Care of the Older Person
A Handbook for Care Assistants

Edited by

Christine McMahon
TD, RGN, BSc, RCNT, RNT

and

Ron Isaacs
RMN, RGN, BA(Hons), Cert Ed

b

Blackwell
Science

© Christine McMahon and Ron Isaacs 1997

Blackwell Science Ltd
Editorial Offices:
Osney Mead, Oxford OX2 0EL
25 John Street, London WC1N 2BL
23 Ainslie Place, Edinburgh EH3 6AJ
238 Main Street, Cambridge
  Massachusetts 02142, USA
54 University Street, Carlton
  Victoria 3053, Australia

Other Editorial Offices:
Arnette Blackwell SA
  224, Boulevard Saint Germain
  75007 Paris, France

Blackwell Wissenschafts-Verlag GmbH
  Kurfürstendamm 57
  10707 Berlin, Germany

  Zehetnergasse 6
  A-1140 Wien
  Austria

First published 1997

Set in 10 on 12pt Souvenir
by DP Photosetting, Aylesbury, Bucks
Printed and bound in Great Britain
at the Alden Press Limited, Oxford and Northampton

The Blackwell Science logo is a trade mark of Blackwell Science
Ltd, registered at the United Kingdom Trade Marks Registry

DISTRIBUTORS

Marston Book Services Ltd
PO Box 269
Abingdon
Oxon OX14 4YN
(*Orders:* Tel: 01235 465500
        Fax: 01235 465555)

USA
  Blackwell Science, Inc.
  238 Main Street
  Cambridge, MA 02142
  (*Orders:* Tel: 800 215-1000
          617 876-7000
        Fax: 617 492-5263)

Canada
  Copp Clark Professional
  200 Adelaide Street, West, 3rd Floor
  Toronto, Ontario M5H 1W7
  (*Orders:* Tel: 416 597-1616
          800 815-9417
        Fax: 416 597-1617)

Australia
  Blackwell Science Pty Ltd
  54 University Street
  Carlton, Victoria 3053
  (*Orders:* Tel: 03 9347-0300
        Fax: 03 9347-5001)

A catalogue record for this title is available from
the British Library

ISBN 0-632-03985-X

Library of Congress
Cataloging-in-Publication Data

Care of the older person: a handbook for care assistants/edited
by Christine McMahon and Ron Isaacs.
    p. cm.
  Includes bibliographical references and index.
  ISBN 0-632-03985-X
  1. Geriatric nursing. 2. Aged – Care. 3. Nursing
assistants. I. McMahon, Christine A. II. Isaacs, Ron.
RC954.C3715 1996
610.73'65–dc20
                                    96-27717
                                        CIP

Contents

List of Contributors

Angela Arnold, *BA*, *RGN*, *OHNC*, *RNT*, Currently working in Occupational Health, with previous experience as co-ordinating, teaching, verifying and assessing vocational qualifications in Care, Assessors and Internal Verifiers awards. Experience in various areas, including food hygiene and safety training.

Kate Arter, *BA(Hons)*, *RGN*, *PGCE*, *RNT*, *TDLB D36*, *32*, *33*, Head of NVQ Development, University of Hertfordshire. Previously established a large assessment centre for NVQs in Care, Assessor and Verifier Awards. Has appeared on BBC television and undertaken Department for Education and Employment projects on access to assessment and APL.

Ruth Ashworth, *BA (Hons)*, *RGN*, *RHV*, *Post Grad Dip in Health Visiting*, *ENB 941*, Primary health care team leader with health visiting responsibilities to 100% Bengali caseload. Previous experience working with older people in both health and social care.

David Bell, *RMN*, Has specialized in working and training carers in dementia care. Currently manages the community nursing services, older people for Riverside Mental Health NHS Trust, London.

David Carpenter, *RMN*, *RGN*, *Dip in Nursing*, *BA(Hons)*, *MA*, Principal lecturer in social philosophy at the University of Portsmouth, specializing in the teaching of ethics, particularly in health care contexts.

Annette Drew, *RGN*, *SCM*, *RNT*, *BSc*, *Diploma in Counselling*, Currently teaching health care assistants and both pre and post registered nurses, specializing in Care of the Older Person. Acts as an Internal Verifier. Experience in the management of residential and nursing homes, with involvement and experience of Vocational Qualifications in Care and Management.

Susan Fell, *RGN*, *ENB 134*, *941*, *998*, *HDQC Physiology*, Currently working as a lecturer in Patient Handling at South Bank University, teaching health care assistants and pre and post registered nurses at University College Hospitals.

Ron Isaacs, *RMN*, *RGN*, *BA (Hons) Cert Ed*, Clinical research nurse. Working for a clinical research and diagnostic service for people with memory problems with the Dementia Research Group, at the National Hospital for Neurology and Neurosurgery, London. Previous experience in specializing in the care of the older person clinically and managerially in hospital settings. Developed and taught on courses concerning care of people with dementia for health and social service professionals.

Christine McMahon, *TD, RGN, BSc, RCNT, RNT* NVQ Consultant training carers. Previous experience as Director Vocational Qualifications, Internal Verifier for Care Awards and Chair of the Royal College of Nursing Vocational Qualification Forum.

James Nash, *BSc (Hons), Dip in Nursing (Lon), RGN, RMN, BTTA, PGCE* Currently teaching health care assistants and pre and post registered nurses, specializing in Mental Health at Bloomsbury and Islington College of Nursing and Midwifery. Has experience in managing the care of the older person, and a special interest in the care of the frail elderly, particularly in relation to healthy ageing.

Jane Powell, *BSc (Hons), Dip in Dietetics, Assessor award (D32/33)* Chief Community Dietitian, this includes areas such as health promotion, training staff and working with housebound clients and their carers.

Helen Souris, *BSc Occupational Therapy* Senior Occupational Therapist working in Mental Health Care of Older People for Camden and Islington Health Authority, based at the Whittington Hospital, London. Has input on the wards as well as in the community – clients' homes, residential and nursing homes.

Jean Valsler, *CQSW, RMN, BA* Experienced nurse and social worker, working with older people in both hospital and community. Involvement in developing and teaching on courses for a wide variety of staff working with older people in both health and social services.

Foreword

Lady Greengross, *OBE*
Director General
Age Concern England

At a time of unprecedented change in the numbers of older people and when new treatments are giving us greater hopes of many more disability-free years, some seemingly intractable problems remain for those who face chronic sickness in later life. They will continue to require skilled care. No group has greater needs and such people are among the most vulnerable and frail in our society. Their needs must be met in a humane and sensitive way which ensures that their lives retain a quality and a sense of enjoyment and fulfilment. Without appropriate and sensitive care, they may simply face more years of dependence and decline than they would have done in the past. For instance, for those suffering from some form of dementia for whom, as memory goes, the experiences of the present become ever more important, a sense of trust, security and love is essential to their well-being. The same applies to all elderly people who depend on others to determine whether their life will retain any quality worthy of that name.

Preparing carers in the different fields of health care for the work they will need to do is an absolute priority. To achieve this aim, a handbook of this style must not only cover caring in the broadest sense, but also provide a knowledge of new interpersonal skills and ways of forming and maintaining relationships.

Care of the Older Person provides essential information for caring for older people in hospitals, residential and nursing homes, in the community and at home. It looks at specialist skills and knowledge, both in supporting sufferers directly and in helping their carers to deal with one of the most difficult situations they will ever face, sometimes over a period of many years. The book provides knowledge of physical health and nutrition, of how to maximize mobility and provide leisure activities, as well as an understanding of ethical issues. These are balanced with a flexible approach combining warmth and personal attention.

I am delighted that this important handbook has been produced. I am sure that *Care of the Older Person* will be very widely read and used as an essential tool for all those caring for older people who need their specialist help and support.

Editors' Acknowledgements

We are grateful to the contributors for their commitment and for sharing their expertise and knowledge for the promotion of a high standard of care of the older person, wherever it may be undertaken.

Our thanks go to Lady Greengross OBE of Age Concern England for writing the Foreword and to all the clients and carers for their assistance and permission to use photographs. Thanks are also due to the Dementia Relief Trust for the photographs in Chapters 2 and 3 and to Lesley Brook for taking the photographs in Chapter 6. In addition, our thanks go to Lorex Synthelabo for permission to use the diagram of the pelvic floor in Chapter 9 and to Jonathan Sichel for the line drawings in Chapter 2.

We also wish to thank our colleagues, Toni Whyman, Mandy Wells, Kenny Gibson and Andrew Day from SLEEPtalk and others who helped to keep us on track to produce a text relevant to the care of the older person and the carers who assist in that care.

We are grateful to Claire McMurtrie and the staff of Blackwell Science for their help and support.

Finally a big thank you to our families and friends for their continual support during the writing of this book, especially Louise for her assistance with the manuscript.

Ron Isaacs
Christine McMahon

About This Book
Christine McMahon

The number of older people in society who rely on care and support from others is increasing. Carers may be relatives, voluntary workers or care assistants and may be looking after the older person at home, in hospital or in a residential or nursing home. Whatever the circumstances, all carers need to acquire the knowledge and skills necessary to deliver care of the highest possible standard. *Care of the Older Person* aims to help them do this by providing the information they need to understand and implement good working practices.

All the contributors to *Care of the Older Person* have specialist knowledge of caring for the older person and have kindly shared their expertise to help produce this book. The general approach is practical and the book provides not only a wealth of information but also numerous descriptions of problems that may be encountered by the carer and suggestions of how best to tackle them. As each chapter is written by an individual you may find the style of writing and level of content varies from chapter to chapter but we feel that this only adds to the overall appeal of the book.

Help with vocational qualifications

The role of the care assistant has developed to support registered practitioners in caring for clients and requires careful direction and supervision by the practitioner. The support offered by care assistants, like any other carer, is enhanced by gaining knowledge and skills through training and many care assistants are now taking the opportunity to obtain vocational qualifications (S/NVQs) which both recognize and develop their skills. This book will help those preparing for assessment for vocational qualifications as it provides the underpinning knowledge needed for a total of 38 units of competence at levels 2 and 3 of the Care awards. An appendix matching up items in the text with the units of the National Occupational Standards for S/NVQs in Care can be found at the back of the book.

A further appendix is provided on accreditation of prior learning (APL) and this will prove of particular interest to those who have been working as care assistants for some years and who have gained considerable skills and knowledge. This experience can be used as evidence to prove competency when undertaking vocational qualifications.

How the book is presented

The book is divided into five major sections. The first introduces some of the general aspects of caring for the older person, and is followed by sections on developing interpersonal skills, promoting independence, assisting activities of living and supporting relatives and other carers looking after older people.

Each chapter begins with an overview and a group of key words which give a brief indication of the contents of the chapter and highlight specific points to be remembered.

Activities

Activities are interspersed throughout the text. These ask you to stop, think and consider what care you would give, or action you would take, under certain circumstances. These *Activities* aim to extend the range of material beyond the text of the chapters and help you use your own thoughts, ideas and experience. You may wish to read the chapter first and then return to the *Activities* later. There is no right or wrong way, whatever you decide to do is right for you.

Do you know?

Throughout the text you will find paragraphs under the heading of *Do you know?* These provide information of additional interest and are intended to help you remember certain items or facts. By the time you have finished the book, and as a result of your own experiences, you may have thought of some *Do you knows?* of your own.

You will also find accounts of specific examples of care given both from the perspective of the client and also from that of the carer. It is hoped that these will give you an insight into the feelings of all concerned in the caring process.

As each chapter is not a definitive work and cannot contain *every* relevant piece of information available, each chapter concludes with a section that provides a list of suggested further reading material and a list of addresses that you may find useful.

The term carer is used to denote the person giving care, such as a relative or a care assistant. The term professional is used to indicate a qualified member of the care team such as a nurse, social worker, physiotherapist, occupational therapist or doctor.

Finally, in order to help you locate the parts of the book you want at any particular time, there is a contents list and a comprehensive index. We hope that you enjoy this book and that you find it complements the care that you give to your older clients.

Section 1
An Introduction

Chapter 1
The Older Person
Ron Isaacs

Overview

The increase in the ageing population highlights the need to appreciate the individuality of the older person. As valued members of society, their rights call for much greater understanding. This chapter looks at the ageing population and its significance for carers. Two contrasting case histories of individual needs of the older person are also identified.

Key words

Stereotypes, rights, independence, valued member, affective disorders, acute confusional state, dementia, prejudices.

Understanding the elderly

Definition

The word 'elderly', another term for the older person, is derived from the word 'elder'. An elder is one who by reason of age or distinction is entrusted with shared authority and leadership which entitles him or her to respect.

Experience of ageing is therefore not uniform, it has no clear boundaries, it is a process that varies from person to person, and will affect all of us at different stages of our lives. Older persons are individuals who are entitled to the same rights, respect, and freedom of choice as any of us. They are valued members of society.

The older person is usually defined as someone aged 60 for women and 65 for men, coinciding with the official age of retirement. As with 'younger' people, the older person's health and welfare will be affected by illness, whether it be of a physical, psychological or social nature.

The prospect of caring for the older person today presents a major challenge. It can be very rewarding and fulfilling and many older people live an active and satisfying life. Others however, experience difficulties as a result of physical infirmity, loss of memory and confusion, which can increase with age.

Do you know?

?

- 4% of the over 65s living at home are bedfast or housebound
- 20% of over 85s living at home are bedfast or housebound
- 30–40% of the over 65s at home have hearing difficulties
- 5% of the over 80s are registered blind
- 16% of women and 8% of men over 75 have regular episodes of urinary incontinence (Rose, 1988)

Those working in acute care, residential, nursing and day care settings will require a greater understanding of the nature of these difficulties, to enable the older person who is in need of care to function adequately and to feel valued in our society.

Stereotypes

The sort of caring we give to the older person need not in any way differ from that of the younger person. This comparison between the young and the old is made in order to dispel unwanted stereotypes that relate to the older person. These stereotypes are concepts which are largely erroneous and if held by a health care worker can seriously affect the delivery of individualized care. Care-giving practices with the elderly require skill, knowledge and aptitude, which when delivered should reflect the needs and personality of that individual. Let us return for a moment to the stereotypes and myths about the older person.

Many carers hold ill-suited beliefs and attitudes of the older person that are inaccurate and inappropriate. (Refer to Chapter 2)

Activity 1.1   ■

From your experience identify the stereotypes and myths held about the older person. For each mentioned discuss with a colleague how it can affect your value judgement, communication and subsequent working practice.

■ ■

Your answers may have included some of the following:

- Many older persons have mobility problems.
- Most older persons do not have similar needs and feelings as ordinary people.
- Most older people are: hard of hearing, slow in their reactions, a burden on society, in need of residential care, irritable.

Failure to perform well is attributed to the well-worn negative cliché 'It's your age'. These are just a few examples of some of the widespread negative stereotype beliefs held by people and are incorrect. It does not help the cause of caring for the older person and this may hinder recruitment of skilled and highly motivated people who may wish to enter this line of work.

Ultimate goal

Over the last few years our knowledge of how to care for the older person is steadily growing. This has led to the creation of new incentives and developments that have been missing for so long.

The ultimate goal is to establish a philosophy of care that will enhance the person's absolute value, whatever the illness or disability. These values should reflect the needs of that person and enable them to live a fulfilling life such as exercising choice, rights, dignity, privacy and independence. This will then set the scene for the establishment of good quality care and practice.

Ageing population

Demographic facts

Pitt (1988) states that, 'Populations age as a consequence of good living standard and public health, low fertility, and improved care of the older person. In the UK, infants survive to be children, children to be adults, adults to be middle aged and the middle aged to be elderly'. We are all growing older by the day and the above statement indicates that we are one and the same person but at different stages of our lives. Each person therefore will have their own individual needs and we as care-givers have an obligation to meet them.

The following figures indicate that the proportion of older people is increasing.

- In 1901, 0.4% of the population was over 75 years old
- In 1981, 6% of the population was over 75 years old (three million)
- In 1981, 0.5% of the population was over 85 years old
- In 1981, 18% of the population of England and Wales were of pensionable age (nine million)
- By 2021, 1.1% of the population will be over 85 years old (Rose, 1988)

One reason for this increase is the baby boom and the saving of young lives at the beginning of this century, along with better health care that enables illnesses to be cured and treated.

Living arrangements

Figure 1.1 indicates that:

Fig. 1.1 Living arrangements of pensioners in 1981.

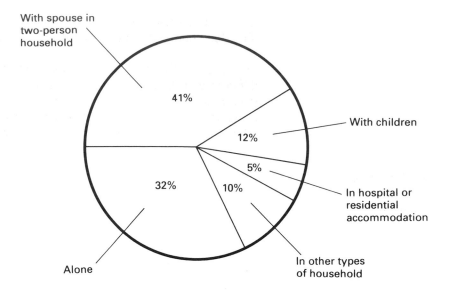

- 41% of older people of pensionable age live with a spouse.
- 32% live alone
- 12% live with children
- 5% are in hospital or residential accommodation and 10% in other types of household (Rose, 1992)

It should be born in mind that this does not necessarily indicate problems of loneliness and subsequent depression.

Some surveys show that about 60% of older people have a son and daughter living within six miles of them; 33% live in the same street or neighbourhood 15% live with a son or daughter. Isolation from sons and daughters is not necessarily a problem for the older person, and a significant number also choose to live alone.

Mental health problems

Health care workers must have an awareness of the mental health problems facing older people. It is important to highlight that mental health problems can occur at any time in one's life for many reasons, and it must not be viewed as a consequence of the ageing process. These mental health problems in the elderly have much in common with psychiatric disorders in adults both in their clinical features and the treatment (Woods & Britton, 1985).

The main classification of illness falls under four main categories

(1) Affective disorders (to include depression and neurosis)
(2) Paraphrenia (schizophrenia in the elderly)

(3) Acute confusional state
(4) Dementia (Alzheimer's Disease and Multi-Infarct Dementia)

The graph in Fig. 1.2 illustrates the number of people with dementia at different ages, these demographic changes indicate that we can no longer ignore the challenge of caring for this group of people. Thankfully we are beginning to make inroads into understanding the nature of dementia and are in a position to develop appropriate skills to meet this challenge.

Fig. 1.2 Epidemiology (source: Dementia Research Group).

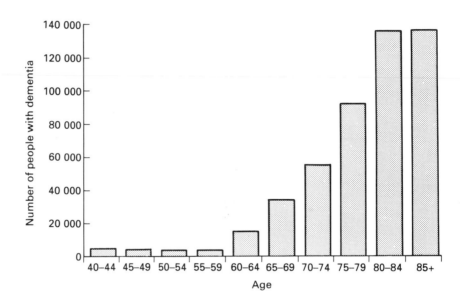

The number of people with dementia in the UK is estimated to be about 600 000. Surveys have shown the prevalence of dementia in the population to be as follows:

Age 40–65   Less that 1 in 1000
    65–70   1 in 50
    70–80   1 in 20
    Over 80   1 in 5
(Source Alzheimer's Disease Society, 1992)

We cannot afford to allow our prejudices to interfere with our work. Working and caring for the older person presents an exciting challenge as advances in care practice steadily improve to meet existing needs; consequently, carers must possess a firm foundation of knowledge and skills.

Here are two contrasting real life examples of the effects of growing old. These provide insight into first the thoughts and feelings of a son reflecting on caring for an aged parent, and second a retired clergyman's thoughts on ageing.

Activity 1.2   ■

Reflect on what the needs would have been for the person in case 1.
Reflect on what the needs would be for the person in case 2 if he was to be
one of your clients.

■ ■

Case study 1
The Effects of Caring for an Aged Parent

Family background
Middle-class parents with one son. Father 15 years older than mother and
son born when father aged 50 years. Mother ceased work when son born
and father retired when son aged 11 years. Family structure such that
mother very much managed the household and undertook all duties
relating to the running of the home. Son married at 23 years, with some
animosity between the father and daughter-in-law. Small family unit with
few close relatives, grandparents having died by 1977.

1982
Mother (aged 62 years) diagnosed as having cancer of the colon which
was treated by surgery. Father found this difficult to accept and dealt with
it by understanding the seriousness of the situation. Caring and support for
the father provided by the son with daily contact whilst mother was hospitalized.

1984
Mother died leaving the father to cope for the first time at age 79 years.
Enormous support needed to try and enable the father to remain living in
the family home with daily contact by the son and meals provided by
neighbours. Cooking, cleaning and clothes washing had all been done by
the mother and now had to be tackled by the father. Night-time dis-
turbances were frequent with the father waking to realize that he was
alone, and when not staying over the son would receive panic phone calls
seeking help. This put a strain on the son's marriage.

1985
Three months after the mother's death, the decision was taken to seek
sheltered accommodation for the father as it was clear that he would
never to be able to cope fully on his own. The animosity between the
father and daughter-in-law increased and placed undue strain on the
son's marriage. A place was secured in a local Abbeyfield home but the
father's grief and depression continued. Night-time calls to the son per-
sisted, many about suicide, and led to a tense atmosphere. Although
physically fit for his age, the father could not accept the loss of his wife
and continued in this way until his death in 1992. The son separated
from his wife in 1991.

Summary

This was a family where it had always been anticipated that the father would die first leaving the mother to cope ably on her own. In the event the circumstances resulted in the grieving of the father for almost seven years and a totally unexpected strain being placed upon the son. Perhaps in the 1990s where so much of the household management is now shared, aged parents will be better prepared to cope with life afterwards.

Case study 2

Retirement at 70 from a lifetime of ministry in the church, including 16 years abroad, brought a sudden and welcome release from the demands of all sorts of responsibilities. Each new day dawned with a glorious sense of freedom, so many pressures were gone and a great sense of space made decision making so much easier.

Of course, there was adjustment to new surroundings and quite unforeseen situations which added to the changing pattern of daily routine. Obligations to the faith at the centre of one's life thankfully remain, but now uncluttered by the claims of parochial administration.

This new-found freedom is like the boost that going into a lower gear gives to an engine, the pace lessens but so does the strain, and this in itself is an enormous relief and source of thankfulness.

The first five years of retirement in a rented flat and looking after myself, were blest with a quiet contentment. One of the greatest blessings was being able to choose what one did each day. This did not mean that there was no ordered pattern in life, but rather that pattern was self-imposed as an expression of the freedom which retirement brings.

Then came an attack of gout, very painful. The left big toe joint turned the colour of beetroot and all but immobilized me but thanks to a guest who was staying with me at the time, I survived, getting to the kitchen was difficult enough, getting to the shops was impossible. I took this to be a warning: a shot across my bows!

The warning was a deep awareness of one's vulnerability with advancing years. I took action and applied for admission to an old established charity and in due time was offered accommodation – please God this will prove to be the last chapter in a long and busy life.

Having a room for one's own use and sharing all meals with some 40 other elderly men, calls for a further readjustment in living. Personally, I have not found this difficult and am happy to say the advantages of care and security by far outweigh the limitations on privacy and personal choice.

One great blessing of living in community is the realization that 'no man is an island unto himself' and if your neighbours' mannerisms and quirks of character irritate you, heaven knows what strain you yourself must be to others! 'Man Know Thyself' is an admonition to heed and act upon every day!

Finally death, a certainty beyond dispute and something to prepare for in one's own mind. Please God at 82 I may accept it, whenever it comes, with penitence for my sins in life, thanksgiving for the privilege of living so long, deep trust in Him who has blessed me throughout my life and will most surely carry me forward to all that lies ahead.

In Case study 1 your answers may have focused on the following:

- The father's bereavement at the loss of his wife leading to his subsequent depression
- The father's sudden change in role reversal by taking over his wife's responsibilities
- The father's reliance on his son's love and devotion
- The conflict between the son and his wife over the father's increasing demand for his son's attention
- The father's lonely existence and the need for companionship

In contrast Case study 2 your answers may reflect the following:

- The self-reliance of a person who demonstrates with determination a strong conviction to his faith.
- This faith of his dominates and guides the way his life is determined. *How do we as carers meet the spiritual needs of our patients?*
- Retirement at 70 years was a happy occasion with a 'glorious sense of freedom'. Other individuals find retirement a difficult and depressing time in their lives. *What are the advantages and disadvantages of retirement?*
- The advantages of care and security for him outweighed the limitations on privacy and personal choice. *What are your views about this and how will it affect the care you give?*

Summary

Caring for the older person demands considerable skill and knowledge. This chapter identifies the need for positive thinking in our caring role and to remember that the needs of each person are unique. The care we give therefore must reflect this principle.

Taking this into consideration our work with the older person should be very rewarding.

References

Pitt, B. (1988) Psychgeriatrics: an overview. *Health Visitor*, August **61**, 247–250.
Rose, N. (1988) *Essential Psychiatry*. Blackwell Science, Oxford.
Woods, R.T. and Britton, P.G. (1985) *Clinical Psychology with the Elderly*. Chapman and Hall, London.

Alzheimer's Disease Society (1992) *The Alzheimer's Disease Report. Caring for Dementia: Today and Tomorrow.* Handel Communications Ltd.

Further reading

Counsel and Care (1995) *Last rights.* Available from counsel and care, Twyman House, 16 Bonny Street, London NW1 9PG.

Kitwood, T. and Benson, S. (1995) *The New Culture of Dementia Care.* Hawker Publications, London.

Holden, U. *et al.* (1995) *Positive Approaches to Dementia Care.* Churchill Livingstone, Edinburgh.

Woods, R.T. (1990) *Alzheimer's Disease.* Souvenir Press, London

Useful addresses

Age Concern England
1268 London Road
London SW16 4ER

Alzheimer's Disease Society
2nd Floor, Gordon House
10 Greencoat Place
London SW1P 1PH

Carers National Association
20–25 Glasshouse Yard
London EC1A 4JS

Dementia Services Development
  Centre
University of Stirling
Stirling FK9 4LA

Help the Aged
16 St. James Walk
Clerkenwell Green
London EC1R 0BE

Social Care Association (Education)
Wrentham House
23 Queens Road
Coventry CV1 3EC

Section 2
Interpersonal Skills

Chapter 2
Communicating with the Older Person
Ron Isaacs

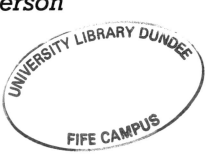

Overview

Effective communication with the older person is of great importance and three main areas will be discussed in this chapter, along with basic guidelines on how to improve communication. First problems of sensory and memory loss will be identified, the consequences of these explored and strategies for managing these difficulties will be discussed. Second, the need to interact with the older person at a time of loss and bereavement will be explored. Finally problems and solutions of aggression will be addressed and how this affects communication.

Key words

Sensory, perception, empathy, self-awareness, warmth, trust, memory loss, dementia, aggression, bereavement, denial, bargaining, acceptance.

What is communication?

Communication can be defined as a process whereby we exchange information and messages through verbal and non-verbal means. This process enables us to share meanings and feelings in an attempt to be understood.

Preconceptions

During an interaction with an older person each will bring to the encounter their own values, experiences, biases, emotions, feelings and attitudes. These factors may influence the understanding of the message and misinterpretation could result. We must employ our sensory skills to perceive and understand the nature of the interaction.

In addition, many obstacles to the way we communicate and interact with the older person can be encountered as a result of:

■ Age, sex, and cultural difference
■ Physical and mental disorders

- Language barriers
- Lack of mutual trust
- Inability to listen and perceive

It is easy to come into a situation or an encounter with preconceived notions of what people are. There is a tendency in society to perceive ageing as a sign of deficiency in the older person. This misconception often leads to poor attitudes towards the older person. The outcome can result in inferior quality of our interaction and communication.

Activity 2.1 ■

From your own experience identify what preconceived notions of the older person are.

■ ■

Your answers may have included such stereotyped views as

- Gerries
- Geriatrics
- Senile

- Unproductive
- Rigid in thought
- Cantankerous

These prejudices can influence the way we perceive an older person and affect the interpersonal relationship. If meaningful communication is to take place then these thoughts and perceptions must change.

Perception is seen as an act of interpreting information which reaches us through our senses. The interpretation may be true or false.

Activity 2.2 ■

Consider the illustration of the 'My wife and my Mother-in-Law' created by cartoonist W.E. Hill and published in the magazines *Puck* in 1915. What do you see?

■ ■

Some of you may see the face of an old woman. Some of you may see the face of a young woman. Some of you may see *both* the old woman and the young woman.

Figure 2.1 tells us that a person can be perceived differently. Our previous experience may have guided the way we select information, but it may also have blinded us to other interpretations. The message therefore is to concentrate on the person and to consider his or her individuality, values and beliefs.

Focus on the person

Everyone needs to communicate. Being understood is the goal of effective communication (Fig 2.2) Understanding another person, whatever their

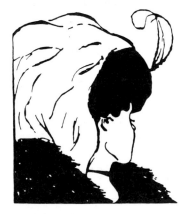

Fig. 2.1 My wife and my mother-in-law.

Fig. 2.2 Focus on the person.

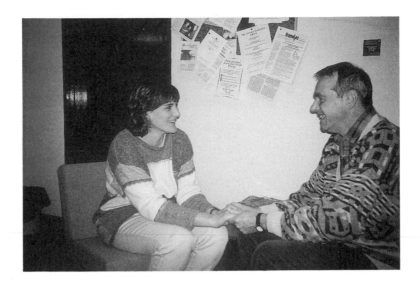

problem, is more difficult than it seems. Therefore it is important to empathize and put yourself *into the place* of that individual. This will help you to understand the older person better and will test your ability to comprehend their world and environment as they perceive it.

Empathy is having the ability to 'sense in oneself the feelings of others' (Eisenberg and Strayer, 1990). Empathy is not the same as sympathy. Sympathy is feeling for, or feeling sorry for, the person. In exercising this approach it will heighten and enhance your skills in communicating, improve the quality of the interaction and establish a good working relationship with the person. This principle of applying empathy in caring should be the hallmark of any form of communication with the older person.

Warmth

In any encounter with an older person it is essential to give them a *warm* welcome. By setting aside all our prejudices the door is open for the expression of warmth, this makes the older person feel equal and secure in a strange environment of a hospital ward, a day centre or a residential home. It builds a feeling of trust between the health care worker and the person.

As we get older physical and mental changes will take place in our lives which may affect our pattern of communication.

Physical changes affecting communication

Activity 2.3 ■

 Make a list of some of the physical, and psycho-social changes which could affect the person's pattern of communication.

■ ■

For physical changes you may have mentioned:

- Hearing disorder
- Visual disorder
- Speech disorder

For psycho-social changes you may have included the following:

- Memory problems
- Confusion
- Bereavement

- Isolation and loneliness
- Depression
- Anxiety

Let us now consider in greater detail how these changes affect communication in the older person.

Hearing Difficulties

Do you know?

?

Hearing is a process which begins with sound. Waves of air which we call sound waves strike at the eardrum. We can neither see nor feel these waves, but the ear is so delicate that the slightest vibration is caught and passed on to the brain. Only when such waves reach the brain do we actually hear. (Leokum, 1978)

There are about 7.5 million people in the UK with some degree of hearing loss and at least three quarters of these people are over 60 years old.

The ear is a delicate organ and can easily be damaged. It has three parts (Fig. 2.3):

Fig. 2.3 Diagram of the ear.

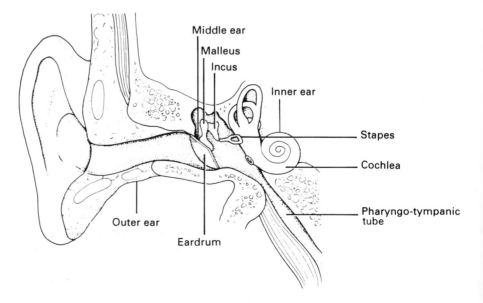

(1) The outer ear: This is the part that is visible and contains the canal which goes down to the ear drum.
(2) The middle ear: This is located at the other side of the ear drum. It contains three tiny bones (Malleus, Incus, Stapes) linked together which move as the ear drum moves in response to sound waves.
(3) The inner ear: This part is very complex. It sorts out all the different sounds so that the brain can receive them.

Damage to any part of the ear, or to the brain can cause deafness. This imposes disruptive barriers to communication and can cause isolation and increase the possibility of depression and paranoia.

Causes of deafness

The most common cause of increasing deafness in older people is *Presbyacusis* (deafness in old age). It is a sensorineural deficit (nerve damage to the inner ear) which reduces the person's ability to hear high pitched sounds, leading to difficulty in discriminating sounds.

Other causes may be due to injury, infection or the side-effects of drugs. The loss may be 'conductive' (inability of the ear to maintain sound transmission) or 'sensorineural'.

Assessment

The most important factor in establishing effective communication with a deaf person is to ascertain the degree of difficulty they have in hearing and to determine the extent of the loss. Some noticeable signs of this may be demonstrated in the following ways. The person may begin to speak in a loud manner when communicating normally. He or she may have difficulty in responding to questions. The older person may be withdrawn, or make an inappropriate response during a conversation.

Communicating with the deaf person

The Royal National Institute for Deaf People has identified 16 points to help the health care worker communicate with the older hard of hearing person.

- Make sure you are in front of and on the same level as the deaf person.
- Position yourself with your face to the light and avoid placing yourself in front of a bright window.
- Check that background noise is kept to a minimum.
- Do not shout.
- Speak clearly, maintaining a normal rhythm of speech.
- Remember that sentences and phrases are easier to understand than isolated words.
- If a word or phrase is not understood, use different words with the same meaning.

- Allow more time for the person to absorb what you have said.
- Keep your head still and stop talking if you turn away.
- Keep hands, pens, etc. away from your face while speaking.
- Do not eat while speaking.
- Avoid exaggerated facial movements, grimacing or inappropriate facial expression.
- Gestures can be helpful.
- If the deaf person is accompanied by a hearing person, avoid conversing only with the hearing person and ignoring the deaf person.
- Make sure the deaf person is looking at you – attract his or her attention if necessary.
- If the topic is changed, make sure the deaf person knows.
- Consult the Standard Manual Alphabet (Fig 2.4).

Fig. 2.4 Standard Manual Alphabet.

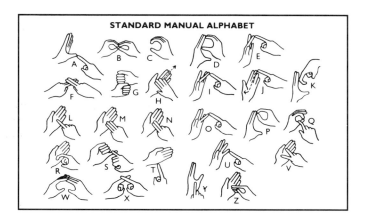

Visual impairment

Do you know?

There are nearly a million blind or partially sighted people in Britain. 66% are aged 75 and over; and about 250 000 live on their own. (RNIB, 1991) (Fig. 2.5)

Causes of visual impairment

Activity 2.4 ■

Make a list of the common causes of visual disability

■ ■

The most common diseases which cause visual impairment are:

- Glaucoma: an increase in raised pressure of fluid in the eye.
- Cataract: degeneration of the lens making it cloudy.

Fig. 2.5 Diagram of the eye.

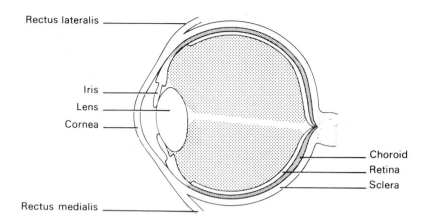

- Diabetic retinopathy: complication of diabetes, bleeding from the retina causing blurred vision.
- Macular degeneration: deterioration of the special cells which enable us to see fine detail.

An interaction, a discourse or an exchange of information is normally initiated by eye contact. Visual signals play an important part in the two-way process of communication, but unfortunately this is absent in the case of the blind person. Someone with visual impairment may have difficulty establishing communication for several reasons.

Activity 2.5 ■

 Why would a blind person have difficulty initiating an interaction while on the ward, a day centre, or a residential home?

■ ■

Your answers may have included these points:

- Feeling a nuisance about having to call out to make a request
- Feeling that the health care worker does not understand a blind person's difficulties
- May avoid contact
- Feeling of being patronized
- Feeling of being prevented from carrying out a task that they are perfectly capable of doing

A person with visual impairment needs to be accepted within the environment. Dialogue and discussion relating to their needs must be identified and responded to.

People who are visually impaired can learn the skills to live in a world full of hazards. These hazards can be minimized by ensuring service delivery is acceptable and appropriate.

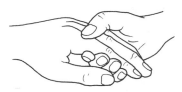

Fig. 2.6 Touching the person.

Communicating effectively

To communicate effectively with someone who is visually impaired and to help them manage safely and independently, the health care worker needs to be aware of the following criteria. Always address the person by name, introduce yourself and ask if assistance is needed. During this introduction touch the person if it is appropriate, so that they are aware of your presence (Fig. 2.6). Often the visually impaired person will hear someone speaking and asking questions, but because there have been no introductions, they sometimes fail to respond. This situation is frustrating and irritating and can be avoided.

When calling on a visually impaired person, check that their environment is free from clutter. The furniture and equipment should remain in the same place and the position of the locker or bedside table is of crucial importance as it usually contains their personal possessions. The person must be informed of any alterations. Make the environment as safe as possible by discarding all objects with sharp edges and creating easily accessible storage space.

Partially sighted people can suffer from light reflecting off surfaces and walls, so try to minimize the glare. To prevent any form of discomfort that can be disabling, there should be curtains at the windows and shiny surfaces should be covered.

When you talk to a visually impaired person, be natural in your conversation using verbal and non-verbal means as appropriate. Position yourself in front of the person and on the same level, with your face to the light and give precise and adequate explanation of any procedures. The person will be relying on the health care worker for guidance.

Activity 2.6 ■

 Are you aware of the organization which can help visually impaired people? It is the Royal National Institute for the Blind, 224 Great Portland Street, London W1N 6AA. Tel: 0171 388 1266. Contact them if you need specific information or advice.

■ ■

Speech difficulties

The speech area is that part of the brain concerned with hearing, speaking, reading and writing. It is situated in the left side of the brain in all people who are right handed and most people who are left-handed. It forms the language system (Fig. 2.7).

The two main areas of the brain concerned with speech are

■ Broca's area
■ Wernicke's area

Fig. 2.7 Language system in the brain.

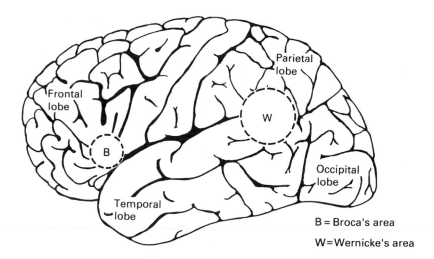

B = Broca's area

W = Wernicke's area

Broca's area is that part of the brain which enables us to organize words for the purpose of producing fluent speech. That area was first described by Dr Paul Broca, a French surgeon. It is situated in the frontal lobe of the brain.

In contrast, Wernicke's area is that part of the brain which allows us to understand and comprehend incoming speech. It was described by Dr Karl Wernicke, a German neurologist. It is situated in the temporal lobe of the brain.

Figure 2.7 shows two areas in proximity to each other. Damage to Broca's area produces problems in articulating words, thus hampering fluent speech. Damage to Wernicke's area will result in failure to understand and comprehend.

Clinical features

Damage to the speech system will produce a defect of speech and language such as:

- Problems in reading and writing
- Inability to produce speech
- Failure to comprehend.

This is commonly referred to as *dysphasia*, and the most common cause is due to a 'stroke' or cerebro-vascular accident (CVA). Other causes of speech disorders are caused by transient ischaemic attacks (TIAs) and tumours of the brain.

Communicating with the speech impaired person

The general principle in meeting the needs of the speech impaired person is to ensure a standard problem-orientated approach which consists of four connecting stages.

(1) Assessment
(2) Planning
(3) Intervention
(4) Evaluation

The *assessment* stage will enable the health care worker to obtain a baseline measurement of the client's abilities to function, including their limitations. The *planning* stage involves identifying specific goals, short and long term to enable the clients to function at their level. *Intervention* involves putting into action the desired goals to meet the needs of the clients. *Evaluating* care involves measuring the effectiveness of your intervention and subsequent outcome. This principle should be applied to any form of care-giving practice including communicating with those who have hearing difficulties and the visually impaired.

An individual assessment of the person with speech impairment may yield the following:

- Need for pen and paper to write
- Need for the carer to be patient
- Need for effective listening skills
- Need to minimize noise
- Need to acknowledge that the person has been understood
- Need to use key words
- Need to use short sentences
- Need to work with the speech therapist

- Need to use verbal and non-verbal means of communication
- Need to involve the relatives
- Need to be aware that the client may become distressed
- Need to give the clients time to express themselves in their own way. Intervene only if you think it is appropriate.

At times there will be difficulties in communicating. To develop a better understanding and more effective way of communicating apply the problem-solving approach as mentioned above and in other parts of this chapter.

Mental and psychological barriers

How do we communicate with the person with dementia?

Do you know?

In 1907 Dr Alois Alzheimer described an unusual dementing illness in a 51 year old woman. She was forgetful, paranoid, and prone to bizarre behaviour. She would get lost even in her own apartment, and would carry objects back and forth and hide them. Her ability to remember was severely disturbed. If one pointed to objects she named most of them correctly, but immediately afterwards she would forget everything again. When reading, she went from one line into another reading the letters or reading with a senseless emphasis. When writing, she repeated individual syllables several times, left out others, and quickly became stranded. When talking, she frequently used perplexing phrases and some paraphrastic (mis-use of words) expressions (e.g. milk-pourer instead of cup). Sometimes one noticed her getting stuck. Some questions she did not comprehend. She seemed no longer to understand the use of some objects ... (Wilkins & Brody, 1969)

That description depicts the striking features of dementia. There were increasing problems with her memory. Her ability to write, read, and speak – the essential component for communicating and interacting – were affected. There were personality changes and socially inappropriate behaviour.

Definition

Dementia can be summarized then as a specific brain disease that results in progressive loss of memory, learning, attention and judgement.

There are many types of dementias, the most common being Alzheimer's disease and Multi-Infarct dementia. The changes most commonly associated with Alzheimer's disease occur in the proteins of the nerve cells in the brain. Under the microscope these changes appear as 'tangles' and 'plaques'. With Multi-Infarct dementia blood supply to small areas of the brain becomes blocked resulting in the tissue dying (infarct). The symptoms for both of these conditions will vary from person to person but they both give rise to progressive impairment of memory and intellectual functions.

Memory loss

The effect of losing one's memory is devastating. Those people who are affected, as those diagnosed with a form of dementia, experience problems in communicating with other people (Fig. 2.8). They often feel worried, anxious, and bewildered when they are unable to:

- Remember the names of familiar objects, people and places
- Do the shopping
- Look up and dial telephone numbers
- Express thoughts
- Travel about in unfamiliar places for fear of getting lost
- Maintain personal interests
- Manage the household finances
- Respond to instructions

As the condition progresses these daily living skills may worsen.

There is a tendency for all of us to avoid those who make us feel uncomfortable. People with memory difficulties, hearing or seeing

Fig. 2.8 Feeling
bewildered.

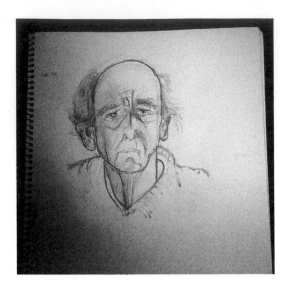

infirmities often present a challenge and can make us feel inadequate as we may find it hard to meet their needs. In situations such as this it is best to try and understand why we wish to avoid contact, to try and remedy the situation. We are probably trying to shield ourselves from the pain and difficulties experienced by these clients. But we must remember that they need communication just like everyone else.

Best care

We care best when we can put ourselves 'in the shoes' of persons with dementia and perceive them as individuals of unconditional self-worth, regardless of their behaviour or difficulties.

Problems in communicating with the person with dementia

Knowing how to communicate with an older person is a challenge. Difficulties occur as a result of memory loss and the inability of the person to process information. These problems arise as a consequence of changes in the brain that control specific memory, language and speech function.

If ignored, individuals are at risk of being socially isolated. Dementia accentuates 'problematic behaviours' and can lead to frustration and anger.

Identify the problem

In your assessment, reflect on the specific difficulty the person is having. The rule is to consider each patient as an individual who has degrees of insight into their illness. It is important to remember that in the early stages of the illness, individuals are aware of their difficulties and try to cover them up.

Activity 2.7 ■■■■■■■■■■■■■■■■■■■■■■■■■

 Make a list of some of the problems which may affect communication with the older person with dementia.

■■■■■■■■■■■■■■■■■■■■■■■■■■■■■

Your list may include some of the following:

- Poor memory
- Repetition of words and phrases
- Impaired word fluency
- Slow response
- Failure to recognize who they are
- Difficulty in writing and reading
- Inability to articulate
- Unable to initiate a conversation

- Reduced vocabulary
- Vague comments
- Says the wrong word
- Has difficulty finding the right word
- Difficulty in naming objects
- Unable to follow instructions
- Repetitive questioning
- Conversation wanders
- Meaningless sentences

We have identified some of the problems persons with dementia experience. The difficulties care-givers face are to respond and to make interaction meaningful.

How to respond

Each situation will be different and the personality of the individual must be taken into consideration. However the following techniques may be useful when planning and agreeing service provision, but on each occasion assess the level of ability of the person before applying these techniques – it may not be appropriate.

Take the lead

Health care workers should respond to remarks and comments in a way that is straightforward. By taking the lead they can control the rate of speech, choice of words, and the amount of information.

Eye contact
This helps the person to focus on you (Fig. 2.9). Be prepared to alter your question. Persons with dementia can experience problems in articulating responses to questions because they cannot find the correct words.

Questions should be phrased in such a way as to cause the least difficulty. To do this avoid open-ended questions, ask questions that limit choices.

Fig. 2.9 Eye contact.

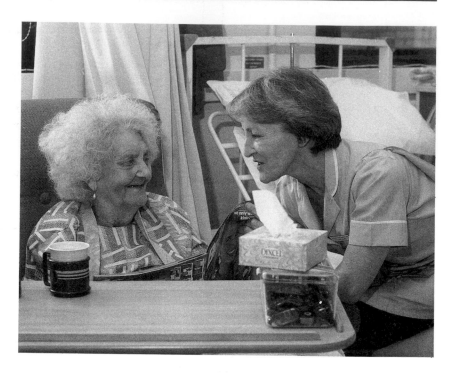

For example: Did you enjoy your holiday? Where did you go? Would you like a drink? Tea or Coffee?

Use key words
Reduce the number of words that are irrelevant, and make the sentence short. Do not include too many thoughts or ideas at any one time. Repeat the key words if necessary.

Give simple instructions
Break the task into simple steps and explain each step before going on to the next. Repeat steps, slowly and clearly while emphazising key words.

Select appropriate topic
Choose topics and conversations that are familiar to the person. In the dialogue you can then modify the discourse, reduce the length of sentence, and use key words for a meaningful interaction. Use different words to express an idea, but keep it simple.

Focus on feeling
Always respond to the emotional feelings of the person. Acknowledge that what is being said may indicate a desire to feel more secure, or that some form of anxiety is being expressed. Work with these feelings.

Look at the facial expression of the client and listen to the tone of voice when these emotions are being expressed, it does give an enormous clue as to how that person is feeling.

Do not ignore the person's attempt to communicate
It is easier to ignore than to engage in an interaction with a person with dementia. This makes the person feel unwanted and a nuisance. Do not agree with comments that you do not understand and which are unreal. Select key words from that comment and focus on them. Reminiscence can enable the person to talk about people and events from the past (see Chapter 12).

Give praise – but do not patronize
It is essential to build a trusting relationship with the person with dementia. This trust will take you further into the interaction and by giving praise, feelings of self-worth and self-esteem will be established. Use touch, if appropriate, to improve the interaction.

Validation approach to care

This was founded by Naomi Feil, a social worker from the USA, and is a way of communicating with the older person with dementia. The word validation means to acknowledge the feelings and emotions of the person and is based on the concept that health care workers are able to communicate with the person with dementia even though the factual content of their conversation is incorrect and 'meaningless'.

It is based on the premise that 'all behaviour has meaning even though it may not always be possible to find out the meaning' (Jones, 1989).

Case study 1

Mrs Clarke, age 72, has been diagnosed as having Alzheimer's disease and has a moderate degree of confusion and memory loss. She has lost much of her language although she can still sing old songs. She is unable to communicate normally. She does however mention words such as 'home', 'mother', 'children' in an otherwise meaningless sentence.

Activity 2.8   ■

How would you respond to Mrs Clarke if during your conversation with her she frequently refers to the past and talks about her home, her mother or the children?

■ ■

The carer can focus on these key words, repeat them back and see if the person can elaborate further. The words 'home', 'mother', 'children' may convey feelings and emotions which Mrs Clarke wishes to express. Acknowledging these facts and empathizing with Mrs Clarke will perhaps enable her to feel secure, safe and less anxious in an environment where communication is encouraged. This approach may not be appropriate for everyone, therefore an adequate assessment of the needs of the individual is important.

Times of stress and loss

Kubler-Ross wrote that:

'Death is usually a natural process, the end to living. Sometimes it is unexpected and sudden – the person goes to bed and dies in his sleep; OR it can follow a long illness and dependence on others.

If death follows a long illness, preparation may be possible both for the family and friends.

We are not very good at talking about death and when we do most of us are ill-prepared. Older people face and will have suffered major losses. Some will have been diagnosed with a terminal illness, others will have lost a close partner, or their ability to hear, see and speak (Kubler-Ross, 1973)

How can we help?

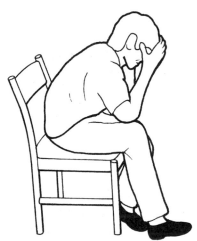

Fig. 2.10 Feeling of loss.

In the event of an older person dying, how can we as health care workers help the client and their family cope with this grieving process? As Kubler-Ross suggests above 'We are not very good at talking about death and when we do most of us are ill-prepared'. All health care workers at some stage in their career will encounter a dying person and grieving relatives and friends.

It is important therefore, that we understand (a) the reaction of someone who has been diagnosed with a terminal illness, (b) the reaction of family members and friends, and (c) our own reaction when it comes to helping clients and relatives cope with bereavement and loss.

Without practice and preparation our attempts to help will often turn out to be tactless and embarrassing. Speaking about major losses and death is not the easiest of activities and as a result the opportunity for useful and helpful interaction is often lost. It is important at this stage to describe the stages of loss and grief as exemplified by Kubler-Ross.

These stages are only a guide to what the person may experience. It is not prescriptive for everyone involved in the grieving process. A flexible approach therefore must be embraced as these stages may not be applicable to everyone.

Activity 2.9 ■

 Reflect on a situation in your life where you have experienced bereavement or loss. What were your reactions and responses to this? Discuss this with your colleagues. Compare and contrast your own feelings with those of a client and the relatives who are experiencing bereavement and loss.

■ ■

Your discussion may have focused on the following points as exemplified by Kubler-Ross in her description of the stages of loss and grief. Consider first the feelings of the client who has a terminal illness and second, the feelings of the relatives.

Denial and isolation

The responses and reactions of many people when told of a diagnosis of a terminal illness may be one of shock, disbelief and numbness. The immediate reaction will be to deny the bad news. 'No, it cannot be true', 'How can this be?', 'It must be a mistake' are some of the responses you may hear. The shock can take the form of physical pain or numbness. Very often the person will isolate themselves, will be feeling scared and may begin to feel sad, lonely and helpless. It is crucial that the health care worker begins to empathize with the person. Allow the person to communicate and vent his or her feelings. Listen to what they have to say and remember it is not always necessary to speak. Speaking about a major loss is not easy and sometimes our responses may be embarrassing and tactless.

Anger

The realization of being faced with a terminal illness may create feelings of anger. This is probably because the client feels frustrated and helpless. The anger may be rational or irrational and may be directed at various people, including the family, doctors and nurses. Some may direct their anger against themselves and may feel resentful and annoyed. This anger is a way of venting feelings of hurt and distress.

Bargaining

During the process the person dying may attempt to postpone death by attempting to tie up loose ends. Some people may want to 'buy more time' by asking their doctor 'how long have I got?'. Others who hold spiritual beliefs may pray for healing or to be given more time. It is very common for the client to begin planning to go places where they have not been before, make amends to people they have offended in the past, or attempt to resolve issues and problems with their family.

Depression

The person may feel depressed as the realization of a terminal illness begins to take hold. They may begin to feel despair, empty or lacking in self-worth and begin to express feelings of:

- Loss of hope
- Loss of confidence
- Misery
- Sorrow
- Guilt

Acceptance

The client gives up the struggle and now faces up to the fears associated with death (Fig. 2.11). Some will come to terms and accept that death is inevitable. However, others may not accept this final decision until the symptoms of the illness increase and begin to affect the quality of their lives. Acceptance will provide comfort for the dying person, but may not always be well received by friends and relatives.

The person is at peace, and may now want to do the things they have always wanted to do. It is important to help them achieve these desires as far as possible. They will make last minute requests to ensure their wishes and desires are fulfilled.

Fig. 2.11 Providing comfort.

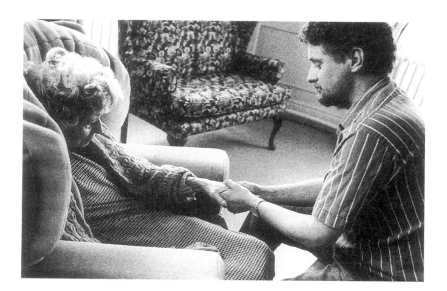

Living bereavement

The term 'living bereavement' is used to describe the experience of loss that occurs when a person develops a dementing illness. The stages of loss and grief as described earlier still apply.

Very often when the client is diagnosed, a major readjustment will take place in the relationship between the client, the spouse and other relatives. This readjustment has to take account of the escalating losses including forgetfulness, communication problems, disorientation, problems with self-care and personality changes.

The client and those close to them will experience the feeling of anger and bitterness. Some will deny the reality of the problem and will hide their feelings. Others may need to express their anxieties and may appreciate professional help.

Whatever the situation, whether clients or families, experiencing a living bereavement, or a conventional bereavement, the need for dialogue is very important if feelings of tremendous isolation are to be avoided.

Supporting the client

Each situation must be viewed on its merits. The above stages will not apply to every person. The sequence may vary therefore it is imperative that the carer assesses each individual situation and responds accordingly. Family support is essential.

The responses you make may be difficult for you to manage, therefore it is important for you to request a senior member of staff to be involved in the interaction. This will help you to build up your experience of preparing to support the older person through grief. This is an emotive and some-times painful interaction, but necessary if help is to be given.

Many people are unable to respond to a dying person or cope with grief expressed by clients and their relatives. This situation can create a barrier to the communication and interaction but it can be avoided. However, being aware of these stages and their implications will enhance your understanding and subsequent interaction.

How to help clients and relatives experiencing loss and bereavement

Allow the subject of death or other reasons for the loss to be discussed. The dying person or those experiencing a loss or living bereavement may wish to discuss practical matters that have been pushed aside. Try to overcome your own discomfort and make an effort to be relaxed in their company and allow them to raise the issue of death and loss. Do not pretend that you can know exactly how they feel. Allow the client to do as much as possible for themselves within their limitations. Being a good listener is very important. Spend time with the client and hear what they are saying. Allow the client to express their guilt and anguish through crying. Some health care workers may feel uncomfortable when someone begins to cry. This is a natural reaction but allow them to release their emotions and feelings.

Managing aggression

Aggression is distressing, hurtful and frightening. It is a cause of great distress to carers and to health care workers. It is a common cause of referral of the person to a hospital or residential home and it can create serious management problems for health care workers.

An understanding of these aggressive acts or problem behaviour exhibited by an older person is crucial to the way it is managed. Therefore communicating effectively between the older person and the carer is essential. Often the reasons for the aggression may be obvious and thus can be solved. But the reasons for aggressive behaviour must be questioned.

What is regarded as aggressive behaviour is by no means straightforward or easy to define. Before any effective management strategy can be implemented, health care workers must attempt to ascertain the underlying cause of the aggressive act and meet it.

Defining what is meant by an aggressive act is open to debate and discussion. The term aggression itself can convey different meanings for different people. Aggressive behaviour must be seen as an overt act involving the delivery of physical or verbal abuse.

Activity 2.10 ■■■■■■■■■■■■■■■■■■■■■■■■■■■■■■

 Drawing on your experience make a list of what you consider to be acts of physical aggression and verbal aggression.

■■■■■■■■■■■■■■■■■■■■■■■■■■■■■■■■■■

Having thought about your answers you may have recorded some of the following:

For physical aggression you may have included these:

- Hitting
- Pulling hair
- Throwing objects
- Pinching
- Scratching

- Kicking
- Biting
- Spitting
- Slapping
- Damaging property

For verbal aggression you may have included these:

- Screaming
- Shouting

- Making verbal threats
- Foul language

These outbursts of physical and aggressive behaviour may have an underlying cause and it is important for health care workers to assess the situation objectively and rule out any misinterpretations and misunderstandings.

Assessing the problem

By assessing the reason for the aggressive act it is then possible to identify the underlying cause: having found the cause, a strategy for solving the problem can be implemented.

Activity 2.11 ■■■■■■■■■■■■■■■■■■■■■■■■■■■■

 For example: Reflect on this situation.

■■■■■■■■■■■■■■■■■■■■■■■■■■■■■■■■■■

Case study 2

Arthur Blake, aged 79, has been living at the Grange residential home for two years. Recently Mr Blake has steadily become incontinent of urine. When the female care assistant attempted to change his (wet) trousers Mr Blake in a fit of anger struck her and began calling her names. The consequences of this aggressive act has led the staff to be very wary of Mr Blake, and a general ill-feeling of suspicion and antagonism exists between him and the staff.

Arthur had never been married. As a young man he pursued a career, in accounting. During the war, he was an officer in the pay corps and following de-mob returned to accountancy. He reached a very high level of management and responsibility for a firm in the City before he retired at 65.

A confirmed bachelor, Arthur was always impeccably dressed and well-groomed; he was always kind and courteous, but stood firm in activities he deemed as being unprincipled. Colleagues remarked on him being over-fussy and somewhat obsessed with being too much of a perfectionist.

He does have poor and deteriorating eyesight. He is also totally deaf in his right ear and needs the use of a hearing aid for his left ear.

Activity 2.12 ■■■■■■■■■■■■■■■■■■■■■■■■■■■■■

Consider possible factors that have contributed to Arthur's aggressive behaviour.

■■■■■■■■■■■■■■■■■■■■■■■■■■■■■■■■■■■■

Problem-solving approach

Adapted from *Understanding Difficult Behaviours* by Robinson, Spencer and White (1989). When you are faced with a difficult situation it is important to analyse and map out the behaviour in order to understand why it occurred.

First of all ask yourself what is the problem? It is evident from the case study that Arthur hit the care giver as she attempted to change his wet clothes. But what precipitated this? There are a number of reasons. Arthur was an intensely private person, and the attempt to change his wet clothes was an affront to his privacy.

Is the patient 'difficult', why?

- Perhaps the carer was too abrupt
- Perhaps she never explained what her intentions were
- Perhaps she made no allowances for his hearing impairments
- Perhaps he could not relate to the carer

The answers to these questions are crucial to the understanding of the problem. Having gained such information about the problem itself consider next:

When does the problem occur?

- Does the aggression take place at mealtimes?
- Does it happen when in the day room?
- Does it occur when in the presence of other people?
- Does it happen suddenly at that time, or is there a precipitating factor?

Who was involved?

- Were there other staff members involved?
- How did they view Mr Blake?
- Was he popular?
- Was he ignored?

Why did it happen?

By gathering the information above, a detailed analysis of the problem of behaviour is mapped out and strategic responses can then be made to solve the difficulties. It is important to look for clues to the cause of the behaviour.

Method of approach

There are no simple solutions but assessing the situation is crucial to good management. Each act of aggression should be assessed on an individual basis as it will be unique to that person. The method of approach will depend on the cause of the behaviour.

In the event of difficult behaviour occurring such as aggression, agitation, incontinence, eating, and wandering, this behaviour analysis programme will provide a helpful instrument when assessing and planning care for the person.

Summary

In this chapter effective communication has been examined along with how it can be accomplished. It has focused specifically on the physical and mental health changes that influences patterns of communication. It presents major challenges to the way we respond to clients and their families and the importance of understanding one another.

By following the suggestions made, health care workers should have greater awareness of the problems of communicating and improve their skills. Furthermore, its application should enhance the dignity, respect, and self-worth of the older person.

References

Burnard, P. (1989) *Teaching Interpersonal Skills*. Chapman and Hall, London.
Burnard, P. (1992) *Learning Human Skills*, Butterworth-Heinemann, Oxford.

Eisenberg, N. & Strayer, J. (1990) *Empathy and its Development.* Cambridge University Press, Cambridge.

Gibson, J. (1981) *Modern Physiology and Anatomy for Nurses.* Blackwell Science, Oxford.

Jones, G. (1989) Caregiving approaches to dementia. *Holistic Health Newsletter*, (22)

Jones, G. & Miesen, B. (1992) *Care-Giving in Dementia.* Routledge, London.

Kubler-Ross, E. (1973) *On Death and Dying.* Macmillan, New York.

Leokum, A. (1978) *Tell Me Why?* Hamlyn, London.

Owens, R. & Naylor, F. (1989) *Living While Dying.* Thorsons Publishers Ltd, Northampton.

RNIB (1991) *Needs Survey.* RNIB, London.

Robinson, A. Spencer, B & White, L. (1989) *Understanding Difficult Behaviours.* Eastern Michigan University.

Rose, N. (1988) *Essential Psychiatry.* Blackwell Science, London.

Shaw, M. (1991) *The Challenge of Ageing.* Churchill Livingstone, London

Wilkins, R.H. & Brody, M.D. (1969) Alzheimer's Disease, *Archives of Neurology*, **21**, 109.

Further reading

Boyer, K. & Watson, R. (1994) A touching story. *Elderly Care*, May/June, **6** (94), 20.

McGregor, I. (1993) Voyage of discovery. *Nursing Times*, 8 September, **89** (36), 29.

Power-Smith, P. (1993) Communal confusion. *Nursing Times*, 8 September, **89** (36), 26.

Smyth, T. (1992) *Caring for Older People.* Macmillan, London.

Stokes, G. (1988) *Aggression.* Winslow Press, Oxford.

Useful addresses

Age Concern England
1268 London Road
London SW16 4ER

Alzheimer's Disease Society
2nd Floor, Gordon House
10 Greencoat Place
London SW1P 1PH

Carers National Association
20–25 Glasshouse Yard
London EC1A 4JS

Cruse Bereavement Care
Cruse House
126 Sheen Road
Richmond
Surrey TW9 1UR

Dementia Services Development
  Centre
University of Stirling
Stirling
FK9 4LA

Royal National Institute for the Blind (RNIB)
224 Great Portland Street
London W1N 6AA

Royal National Institute for the Deaf
19–23 Heatherstone Street
London EC1Y 8SL
Tel: 0171 296 8000

Chapter 3
Relationships and the Older Person
James Nash

Overview

Human relationships are central and essential to both the physical and sociological functioning of the older person. Repeated surveys of older people asking them to name factors that are most important in their life find relationships figure predominately, with health as a significant issue of their lives. This chapter will examine relationships in their widest context, including sexual relationships. Relationships in this client group are important and will be considered as part of the broad picture. Also this chapter will discuss how carers can facilitate and enhance relationships with clients, recognizing in the process how relationships can promote self-esteem, mental and physical health and a state of wellness with clients.

Key words

Confusion, dementia, depression, empowerment, ethic, exercise, privacy, relationships, reality orientation, self-esteem, sexuality, social isolation, wellness.

Social background and the older person

The demographic representation of older people in society has been examined by Jacques (1995) who provides the following statistics. In Britain 15.8% of the population was aged 65 years in 1991. With the advancing years the male to female ratio falls steadily from 1:1.2 in the 65–69 year age group to 1:3.0 in the 85 years plus age group. As a result, older women find themselves increasingly alone. Only 5% of the total elderly population in Britain lives in institutional care. While 15% of the elderly experience a serious psychiatric problem, consequently psychiatric illness in the elderly tends to be a community problem. The major causes of mental and physical ill health in the later years of life are very often multi-factorial in origin. Both social and physical factors have been implicated as contributory towards the psychopathology, these include:

- Poverty and economic disadvantage.
- A poor nutritional state.

- Loss of physical integrity, for example, failing eyesight and deafness, resulting in increased sensory deprivation.
- Social isolation.
- The experience of repeated loss, the loss of paid employment and work-related social networks due to retirement. In relationships, the loss of a partner and friends with the resulting constant attendant pain of bereavement. The possible losses of social involvement, parental role, physical and mental agility and the loss of an opinion making role.

Isolation

Social isolation and sensory deprivation may result in the older person becoming apathetic, confused, indifferent, depressed, fearful and paranoid. Which in turn can result in mental illness and in increased health costs. Garrett (1991) reminds us that the older person's body image, sexual and interpersonal relationships can be changed by surgical procedures like mastectomy, stoma creation and amputation. While other disabilities like arthritis, heart attack, urinary incontinence and stroke may profoundly affect how the older person views themselves. Feelings of loss of self-worth and value may occur accompanied by a withdrawal from social interaction. Older people are often living alone and excluded from the main activity in society and in the process they become disempowered.

Activity 3.1 ■

You are watching the television evening news programme. Individuals are seen demonstrating against a recent government proposal, among the demonstrators are several older persons. What do you think would be your first impressions and feelings on seeing older people?

■ ■

Your answer may have been: 'Good for them standing up for what they believe in' or, 'They are old enough to know better, causing trouble at their age'. The answer most likely to occur is, 'I did not notice older persons in the demonstration'. This shows the kind of 'invisibility' older persons often experience.

Whether or not you agree with the demonstrators and their views is of course immaterial. What you would have been observing, had you noticed, was older persons actively involved in social and political relationships. For most older persons even though the process of ageing may slow them down, they remain comparatively fit and independent, sometimes to the end of their lives. Throughout this time many older persons continue to engage in both purposeful and meaningful relationships, however this may not always be the case.

Disempowerment and the older person

Disempowerment tends to take two principal forms.

Social disempowerment

With social disempowerment the individual is gradually excluded from social activity resulting from traditional changes in the social structure of their life. The loss of work due to retirement or redundancy, a corresponding decline in economic spending power, children leaving the parental home to forge their own way in the world, are just a few of the changes. Social marginalization of the older person devalues the continued contribution that they can make to the function and progress of society.

Personal disempowerment

The older person may disempower themselves. They often comply with the way society expects them to perform the stereotyped role of the older person. They adopt the attitude and behaviour of not wanting to make a fuss, of being grateful for any consideration shown to them. Gradually and imperceptibly the older person disengages from the political and social scene. Withdrawal from social interaction occurs. The older person begins to acquiesce in their own decline. Very often health care workers will encourage this attitude. The compliant client is easier to care for and, as a result, the carer may inadvertently contribute to the older person's disempowerment, agreeing all too frequently with clients when they say, 'Well it's my age, the doctor said' or, 'I am not as strong as I used to be' or, 'I do not get out much'. Both carer and client may contribute to the client's loss of independence. In addition both parties may promote the stereotypical ageist views. The concept of ageism defines the older person as a member of a homogeneous group, sexless, senile, inferior, past making a valued contribution, physically decrepit, mentally slow and a passive, helpless victim. To overcome this bias, we need to look at relationships and how they work.

Taking a closer look at relationships

Activity 3.2 ■

 What are the most important aspects in a relationship to you? Write down a list of what you consider to be of value in your own personal relationships and why?

■ ■

Some examples you may have included in your own list may be:

■ Trust. Because it provides reliability, strength and confidence in a relationship.

■ Honesty. Because it provides sincerity and genuineness in a relationship.

■ Friendship. Because that person will spend time with you, they are sympathetic, non-threatening, supportive, they know your faults, but never judge you. You are loved and cared for in a non-sexual way.

■ Companionship. Because being together means you can relax, you can share interests, ideas, values and beliefs in common, it prevents loneliness and feelings of isolation.

Other points on your list may include: love, emotional support and the opportunity to engage in shared struggles and shared laughter, pain and pleasure.

Client and carer relationships

The relationship which exists between a client and health care worker (carer) in many ways contains similarities to other personal relationships, containing the above aspects and yet in many ways is markedly different. The relationship is an interpersonal one. Gross (1987) who has looked at the subject of relationships, describes how relationships need to be rewarding. They are influenced by degrees of compatibility between two people such as education, age, emotional and physical attractiveness. Other influences include the relationship of the person with the carer, the amount of times the carer sees the person, and the level of familiarity. When the client and carer share similar values, the client's self-esteem increases with acceptance, and communication is easier (Fig. 3.1). How-

Fig. 3.1 Friendship.

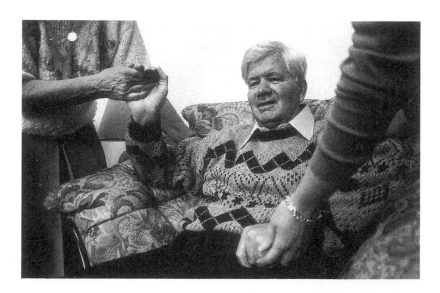

ever, clients and carers may not choose one another, so what should happen to promote a rewarding relationship?

Core values

The core values of a relationship need to be recognized. These include demonstrating respect for the client's

- Ethnic origin
- Values
- Attitudes
- Religious beliefs

- Past learning
- Life experiences
- Sexual orientation
- Opinions

This does not mean that you have to agree with everything the client may say or do. Nor does it mean colluding with a client's prejudice and bigotry, or expecting the client to always agree with you. It means recognizing the client's right to have their own ideas and thoughts and recognizing the integrity of the individual. The client should not be exploited, humiliated or ridiculed and should not be taken advantage of either physically, emotionally or financially (see Chapter 6 Elder Abuse).

Carers' relationships with the older person

The most difficult aspect of the health care worker's relationship with a client is trying to maintain an appropriate level of intimacy. Maintaining a successful relationship with a client will often depend on how that relationship is managed. In caring for the older person it can be very easy to become over familiar, to treat the older person in a child-like fashion, to become regimented in the approach to care-giving. All too often the older person may experience depersonalization from carers. The client's personal space may be invaded without prior consent and should the client protest they may be labelled as 'difficult', 'unpopular' or 'awkward' by carers.

The level of intimacy between a client and a carer in a relationship will be influenced by many aspects including;

- Age
- Sex
- Personality

- Ethnic origin
- Education and cultural background

It is useful to remember however that the evidence has repeatedly demonstrated that women move to a deeper level of intimacy in relationships much faster than men. This gender difference can mean the older adult male may be suspicious or resentful if the carer tries to establish a relationship with too great a level of intimacy too soon. While for the older female when the relationship moves to an intimate level too fast her rights of privacy and respect may be compromised inadvertently by carers. The relationship between a client and carer has dynamic power. The balance of that power needs to be constantly shifted in favour of the client to allow them to act with autonomy and independence.

Managing a relationship with an older person

The personality and character of the older person can remain consistent as ageing increases. However, the conceptual boundaries change. The older person is often more introspective, cautious and reflective about their life and looking back at past events. The older person is often less spontaneous in thought and behaviour. Reminiscence of their life's events can provoke powerful memories of happy and sad periods which stimulate feelings of joy and contentment, or disappointment, remembered failure and despair. During a period of illness the older person can often be unduly pessimistic, concentrating on negative aspects of their life, so that self-esteem and self-worth are undermined. As a result the subsequent recovery may be impaired. The way a carer establishes and manages a relationship with a client can profoundly influence the recovery outcome.

At this period in a client's care, the carer has the opportunity to act as both a friend and as a change agent for the client. The carer becomes an instrument which is part of the therapeutic process. What can the carer do?

Guidelines in the relationship with an older person

Always ensure the relationship operates within the boundaries of the law.

Empower clients whenever possible to make and take their own decisions when providing care and allow the client the right to control their own environment.

Provide a clear rationale for the delivery of care. In other words, explain clearly why certain procedures, tests and treatments are necessary and why certain nursing action is required. Always respect the client's right to confidentiality, privacy and feelings of independence. In the process, build a positive relationship with the client, demonstrating respect for the client's life experience and previous learning.

Assess the client's strengths and resources, their autonomy, thinking ability, flexibility and spirituality. Concentrate on their strengths. Recognize their problem-solving skills. Compliment them on their appearance and the effort they make to use effective strategies for coping.

Assess the client's external resources, such as their partners or other members of the family. Also assess other members of the caring team and support networks. In short, all those who can provide assistance to the client's advantage.

Develop a relationship which embraces, provides comfort, maintains honesty, fosters trust and conveys a positive attitude.

Personal growth continues throughout life, so encourage the older person to concentrate on the best aspects of their life. If the client has worked, raised a family, cared for an aged parent, taken an interest in the future for young people, the environment, the state of the world and social justice, these are positive issues in a person's life. They demonstrate commitment and motivation. The use of praise and adopting a sincere attitude with a client in the course of social interaction will add purpose and meaning to a client's life and assist in their continued journey toward self-discovery.

Social relationships

As a friend, carer and change agent you are participating in a therapeutic endeavour. The value of the social relationship that you engage in will enhance a client's life, increasing a sense of:

- Social well-being
- Improved mental health
- Improved physical health

The benefits of social relationships have been shown to relieve and to reduce stress. They increase self-esteem and self-confidence and lead to an improved all-round health status. Good social interactions have been recognized as being part of:

- Reducing feelings of depression and isolation
- Reducing feelings of worry and anxiety
- Providing support in times of difficulty
- Enhancing the recovery from illness

Through the befriending relationship, hope is established once again. As Forbes (1994) states the older person is helped to adapt and to transcend the normal ageing process. A realistic perspective is engendered. The older person is empowered, encouraged and renewed. Feelings of powerlessness and hopelessness are overcome. The provision of active listening will give the client the opportunity to reminisce, to vent feelings of anger and disappointment in a safe environment. Through the befriending relationship the client will feel less lonely and gradually any disturbance to the individual's personal identity is given a chance to make a healthy adjustment (see Chapter 2, Communications).

Activity 3.3 ■

So far we have considered relationships where the client is willing to engage in social interaction with a carer. This is often not the case. Write down a short list of your feelings when a client refuses to engage in a social relationship with you and may even be hostile or actively aggressive. How do you feel?

■ ■

On your list of feelings you may have included:

- Hurt
- Anger
- Confusion

- Bewilderment
- Hopelessness

You may feel hostile and aggressive in return, other feelings may include a sense of rejection, physical pain and you may take avoidance behaviour. In addition, you may call into question your own worth, and very often job satisfaction is also questioned. You have a right to your feelings and acknowledging them is the first step in building a relationship with a difficult client.

Coping with difficult older people

For some older persons their experience of close relationships in life may have caused them pain. They may have invested a great deal in a marriage, only for it to end in divorce. Or they may have invested all their energy in a job, only to be constantly unsuccessful when seeking promotion, or be made redundant.

Events such as the death of a child or a partner, may have left the older person damaged. The individual's past experiences in relationships could mean the risk of future commitment is viewed with alarm. Past experiences of social breakdown in previous human relationships in the client's life may have resulted in feelings of worthlessness and demoralization. The client may perceive themselves to be unattractive.

Increased anxiety is often expressed by clients who fear further loss of independence or resent increased feelings of vulnerability when being cared for. Before a client's aggression and hostility results in them being labelled a 'difficult client' it is important to keep in mind that aggression and hostile behaviour from an older person has a purpose. It may be:

- A self-protection mechanism against a perceived threat
- Providing the individual with a measure of control in a strange, uncertain environment
- A response to stress
- A means of self-preservation
- A means of increasing self-esteem and self-worth
- Protecting the client against increased vulnerability

Positive approach to care

How then should the carer act? Faced with apparent anti-social behaviour the carer should not respond or act in negative way, but remain calm. Do not engage in a destructive dialogue with other staff about the client's behaviour, instead try to understand why the client is acting in this way. Set the behaviour in context to the client's view of life. Always let the client know they are valued and continue to act with warmth, empathy and genuineness. Do not ridicule or trivialize the client's distress. The responsibilities of the carer to the client remain identical to those where clients are co-operative. However, you do have the right to say you are hurt and upset by their behaviour.

In the course of your caring relationship with the client you may be having a very positive effect. The overall objective is to reduce stress and to strive to improve social relationships for the client. But it may take much longer to reach that point where the relationship is a relaxed and a comfortable one for both of you. On the other hand, you may have to accept you may never be privileged to know the value of the relationship you have with a client. The client may be unable to reciprocate friendship and may be unable to feel comfortable with or trust self disclosure to you. But this in no way devalues the effort made by carers in the befriending relationship.

Sexual relationships and the older person

The area in human relationships that remains the most contentious is that of sexual relationships. For the older adult, expressing their sexuality is often viewed as a joke or even worse, ignored. The subject is surrounded by stigma. As a consequence, an older person requiring help in their sexual relationship is reluctant to ask for it. The problem then is hidden by default. Masters & Johnson (1966) demonstrated quite conclusively that the older person is capable of sexual expression, enjoyment and pleasure right into the eighth decade of life. Sexual problems in the older person are very frequently associated with the ageing process, but by no means exclusively so. Sexual dysfunction is often caused by factors that are not directly related to the ability to perform the act of sexual intercourse. Factors include:

- Anxiety
- A misunderstanding between a couple
- Low self-esteem
- Mental and physical frailty
- Stress
- Depression
- Overeating and drinking
- Illness
- An unsuitable environment, noise, distractions and a lack of privacy
- Reduced opportunity
- The negative attitude of carers and ageist attitudes

Recognition that older people have a capability to enjoy an active sex life is to acknowledge their right to sexual health services. For the older person who is not in a monogamous sexual relationship and engages in casual sex or who may purchase commercial sex, the need to provide them with sexual health advice is important. This will include a regular sexual health check-up to exclude the potential risk of having acquired a sexually transmitted disease. The client will also require education and advice on safer sex practices, plus the client will need to understand their sexual risk behaviours. This education takes time. If carers are unsympathetic to the sexual health of older clients, they may be unable to feel confident in accessing the service provision. Promoting sexual health and healthy sexual function in older people is part of the total care management.

Physical changes in sexual function

In general, as the individual ages changes take place in sexual response. In the older male penile erection takes longer to occur. More direct stimulation is often needed initially to achieve an erection. Ejaculation is reduced in intensity and in frequency. In the older female pain experienced during sexual intercourse is very common due to inadequate vaginal lubrication. The vagina becomes narrower and shorter and the clitoris decreases in size. These physical changes are not insurmountable. Providing an explanation of the physical changes and the use of water-soluble lubricants will reduce anxiety. Very often in this client group education about alternative sexual techniques and positions is of help to those who suffer from respiratory, or cardiac disease and reduced mobility from arthritis. The important point is for the carer to adopt a positive attitude to the client's difficulties and to be able to refer to the appropriate person for help. This could be a doctor, psychologist or a nurse specialist.

The older adult female and male homosexual

The older homosexual may face prejudicial views toward their sexual orientation and stereotypical ageist attitudes. Many older gay men will remember a time when male homosexuality was classified as a psychiatric disorder and the act of consenting sexual intercourse with another adult male was illegal. This is still felt, despite changes in the law and a greater social acceptance of alternative life-styles and the acknowledgment of sexual diversity. Many older male and female homosexuals are still uneasy with their sexual identity. This may mean they remain isolated and secretive about their sexual orientation. They may be fearful, anxious or uncomfortable with disclosure.

In the UK the more radical high profile, political stance of the younger members of the gay community has not yet completely embraced the older members of the community. In the USA the situation is slightly different. The older homosexual has a far more socially visible presence. Role models are more in evidence, with such groups as 'The Older Homosexual in the Environment'. Being grey and gay has a more positive perspective and their history and life experiences are being assiduously recorded and valued. As the younger members of the gay community carry their sexual politics into middle and old age it is reasonable to speculate that the situation will change for homosexual older people in the UK. Service provision will change to meet their later life needs.

Relationships with older homosexuals

If the older person in the course of being cared for discloses their sexual orientation to you or you recognize they have a loving partner of the same sex. What can you do? Homosexual men and women do not expect special treatment or rights. They do expect and deserve equal rights, confidentiality and respect. Carers need to recognize that for them growing up gay was a very different life experience than it is today. Often before the amendment to the criminal law male homosexual relationships were furtive, secretive and even dangerous. While lesbian relationships have never been illegal, for older lesbians the relationships were subject to social disapproval and condemnation.

Older homosexuals may still view themselves as social outcasts. In an attempt to fit in with society and in an effort to secure love and affection, they may have compromised who they really are. In the later years of life this can contribute to ill health, feelings of resentment, that the true self was suppressed or denied.

Positive approach to homosexuality

Encourage the older homosexual to be:

- Positive about their life, even its difficulties.
- Reinforce the client's sexuality in a positive way.
- Do not threaten, humiliate or dismiss a client's sexuality or use abusive names to describe it.
- Demonstrate a relaxed attitude to the client's sexual orientation.
- Encourage the client to express their feelings in relation to their sexual orientation.
- Reinforce for the client the positive aspects that have taken place in the wider society that have benefited gay men and women.
- Acknowledge the client's right to express their sexuality.
- Try to identify any care needs that may be needed for this particular client group. These include the need for privacy or an opportunity to access particular services.

The older homosexual will benefit from maintaining relationships with friends and being encouraged to develop new friendships. Caroline (1993) has described friendship as 'a meaningful and highly significant human activity'.

Ask the client if they require help from the gay community organizations. For example, the gay befriending groups or gay bereavement support and counselling services. In addition, the client may appreciate access to books documenting the struggle, feelings and life histories of gay men and women. This may help the client see their own life in some perspective and reduce feelings of alienation.

Homosexuals are not a homogeneous minority group. The diversity in the homosexual community is as varied as for heterosexuals, so care provision needs to be designed on an individual assessment of needs.

Expressing sexuality in relationships

Activity 3.4   ■

Sexual intercourse and sexual identity are just two ways in which sexuality is expressed. Consider other ways that individuals may express their sexuality.

■ ■

Having considered the question, you probably realize that individuals express their sexuality in all areas of their lives such as:

- Behaviour
- The way a person moves
- Personality

- Appearance and dress
- Choice of books they read and the music they listen to

Almost all aspects of an individual's life is concerned with sexual expression. *Sex* is biologically determined – an individual is either male or female. *Gender* is a socially defined concept, consisting of masculine and feminine. The gender stereotyping of individuals can be the cause of much unhappiness. For example, men are expected to be active, assertive and competitive. They are expected to avoid emotional, demonstrative behaviour and to display both physical and psychological strength. Women are categorized as talkative, gentle, neat in appearance and habits. Women also tend to be viewed as submissive in nature and more psychologically fragile. Gender is not an absolute concept. It varies over time and between societies and within the same society. However, so powerful is its influence, it can often prevent or spoil relationships as individuals struggle to conform to the role expected of them. This is reinforced by society, family, peers and friends. Clients who express their sexuality differently from the gender assigned role may be subjected to unsympathetic attitudes from carers. The older female client who is assertive, informed and demonstrates strong coping strategies may be viewed as hard and unfeminine. Carers may form a prejudical attitude toward her expression of sexuality.

Attitudes concern a person's likes and dislikes. They are expressed in:

- What you think
- What you say

- What you feel
- The way you behave

A *prejudice* is described as an extreme attitude.

Looks and appearance

Expressing sexuality is often an unconscious process. Some clients and carers may be very physical in their approach to others. They may stand very close in a confidential manner and engage in a lot of touching during a conversation. Others are more reserved, with a preference for maintaining space between themselves and the other person and rarely touch or embrace others. The older person can often be very particular about their appearance. For many women, the clothes they wear, their make-up and hair style are integral to the way they view themselves. While many older men feel only semi-dressed if they are not wearing a tie or waistcoat. Often, the older male has a regular routine for getting his hair cut (see Chapter 10). Clients also express their sexuality in the surrounding environment. Some residential nursing homes recognize this need and allow clients the opportunity to bring with them personal possessions like bed covers, small items of furniture to display books or china collection and pictures to hang on the wall.

Expressing sexuality within the care environment

The older person is cared for in a variety of care environments. These include hospitals, private and local authority nursing homes and the patient's own home. The opportunity for older people to express their sexuality will be influenced by:

- Sensitivity of the staff
- Resources available to the organization
- Organizational management
- Other residents, neighbours and family
- Client's freedom, mobility and personal finances

irrespective of the context in which a client is cared for. Enabling an individual to express their sexuality, using the term in its widest interpretation, can be a creative and life enhancing force which substantially benefits clients' lives.

Activity 3.5 ■

 Now take a moment to reflect, to think about your own sexuality. Do you feel comfortable with the topic? Write down a short paragraph describing yourself and your attitude to the subject of sexuality.

■ ■

Your own sexuality

Whatever you have written is confidential to you alone. Why is it important? Let us take an example. Would you describe yourself as a sentimental person? Many clients are, they often attach considerable affection to a particular object, possibly a ring or photograph. For clients to feel comfortable expressing their sexuality, carers need to feel confident and have a self-awareness of their own sexuality. Recognizing that you are quite possibly not a sentimental person, and being comfortable with that perspective, will give you insight to respect and value any sentimentality exhibited by clients. Knowing yourself, acknowledging your attitudes and feelings and being able to admit to them will foster mature relationships with clients and promote independence, growth and wellness in clients. It will also enable you to communicate more effectively in a relaxed and friendly way in relationships.

Promoting wellness

A working definition

Promoting wellness can be described as using health promotion within the caring relationship. It enables the older person to feel physically and psychologically comfortable with themselves, irrespective of any disease process or decline due to the natural ageing process. The carer's relationship with the client is used to facilitate this objective.

Factors promoting wellness

In her discussion on promoting wellness in older people Miller (1991) has identified several factors that can enable the carer to help clients. These included a whole host of attributes that are very often intrinsic to the client.
  Factors offering health protectiveness included:

- *Relationships*. The larger the network of relationships the older person had the greater health protectiveness they provided.
- *Altruism*. This was identified as a health protecting factor, the demonstration of concern and care for one's fellow man.
- *Resilience*. This means older people who demonstrated the ability to fight and bounce back in adversity.
- *Hardiness*. This was described as the ability to take a firm stand and exhibit courage in the face of life's difficulties.
- *Global concern*. This was the continued ability to express concern for the welfare of the planet and the environment, such as campaigning against pollution and ecological damage.
- *Personal growth*. This was the recognition that the ageing process was part of the human growth pattern, not something to be marginalized and feared.

- *Diet and exercise.* The eating of a well-balanced nutritional diet and continuing to take regular exercise was seen as positive to protecting health (see Chapters 8, 11 and 12). Shephard (1990) supports the role of exercise in the older person. No matter how old the client is, a prescribed exercise program will add 'quality of life by maximizing residual function'.

Self-care

Using the findings identified by Miller (1991) it is possible for carers to help clients by assisting in their independence. Carers can also promote self-care and not restrict the older person's opportunity to take on continuing self-responsibility. The carer is able to recognize the older person's strengths and use them to promote a state of wellness, supporting the client with praise and respect.

The older person can be helped to adapt past learning skills to new situations; to formulate new hobbies and interests and modify old ones. Relationships need to be preserved with family, friends and newer social networks can be developed. The role that a carer plays in the client's life is crucial to promoting wellness. Two issues have been identified by Miller as being important, they are: the opportunity for older people to continue with activities and to enjoy relationships of their own choice.

Activity 3.6 ■■■■■■■■■■■■■■■■■■■■■■■■■

 What sort of carer are you? Write down a short list of the aspects of caring that are important to you when caring for an older person.

■■■■■■■■■■■■■■■■■■■■■■■■■■■■■■■■

Empower your client

With this activity you will be able to demonstrate how you approach the activity of caring.

- Do you let clients take risks?
- Are you the sort of carer who likes to do things for people?
- Do you take time to sit and talk to clients?
- Do you take an active interest in helping them to help themselves?

Knowing what sort of carer you are and your approach to caring will help you identify your own strengths and where you may need to modify or change your stance. It is very hard to stand back and let clients do things for themselves. But often carers need to make adjustments if clients are to benefit. Old age is a culturally defined concept and with the concept goes a variety of false ideas such as:

- Older people are in need of constant help
- Older people do not have sex
- Older people find it hard to learn new things

Older people are subject to stereotyping, learned helplessness and disempowerment. The statements about them are often myths. In fact older people are amazing. A political and social force of considerable strength, whose number looks to increase substantially in the future.

Relationships with the vulnerable

In our discussion on maintaining relationships with older people so far, we have concentrated on the older person who has to some extent the ability to engage in a relationship with a carer. We now turn our attention to the most vulnerable of older people. This client group whose dependency and fragility requires the carer to act with absolute integrity when maintaining relationships.

The vulnerable older person includes those who are confused and clients suffering from dementia. Scrutton (1989) who has looked at the subject of confusion in the older person, points out that very often confusion is a subjective value judgement. He has argued that it has been estimated that between 5 and 10% older people suffer from confusion and the numbers are on the increase. Confusion is not a normal feature of ageing, but it is often assumed to be the case.

Assessment of the confused client

Whatever the cause, Mathieson *et al.* (1994) recommend the carer should first make an assessment of the client's confused state. This will enable the carer to provide the most appropriate care. An idea of the client's recent history is required. The sort information you need to know includes:

(1) Have the changes to the client's mental state occurred gradually, or has it been sudden?
(2) What sort of symptoms have been demonstrated by the client in the confused state that were not present before?
(3) Is the confusion worse at any particular time of day?
(4) Has the client had a recent illness or operation and is he or she on any medication? If so what is it?
(5) What is the client's normal mental state like?
(6) What type of memory loss is the client experiencing? Is it a loss of recent memory or past, distant memory, or both?
(7) At the same time an assessment is needed of the client's level of consciousness. This involves their thought processes and the clarity and content of their speech.

(8) An assessment also is needed of the client's perception of reality. Is the client aware of their surroundings? Do they know who you are, the time of day, the year and the season?

(9) The carer also needs to be aware of the client's functional abilities. This will comprise all the activities that are involved in daily living. Activities include, washing, bathing, continence, using the toilet, eating, drinking and mobility.

Irrespective of whether the client's confused state is temporary or progressive, the way a carer maintains a relationship with a client will have an impact on the client's confusion.

Caring for a confused, vulnerable older person

Two aspects of the carer's approach to the management of a confused client are very important, these are:

(1) The way a carer manages their own behaviour when carrying out their duties

(2) The carer's powers of observation

If the carer is rushed, anxious and disorganized or loud in their speech and gives too many instructions to the client, this will aggravate the client's confused state of mind. The carer's behavioural approach to a confused client needs to be one that promotes a sense of quiet and calm. Focus on the client directly, maintain eye contact, use a reassuring facial expression. Keep instructions to a minimum. Make those instructions clear and unambivalent with preferably only a 'yes' or 'no' answer being required.

Observation of a client's behaviour will enable you to be able to identify any stress in the client's environment liable to increase the client's confused state. For example, if a client starts to run and open doors then looks anxious or starts to cry before being incontinent, he or she is probably looking for the toilet.

Sexual expression and confusion

Two challenging behaviours that cause the most distress are an inappropriate sexual expression and wandering. In order to help a confused client it is necessary for the carer to *place the client's behaviour within a context. This means trying to understand what the client is thinking at the time.*

The client may be experiencing time confusion that results in wandering. For example, they may think of themselves as young again and attempt to go to work. Sexual behaviour may be expressed as a basic human need. Or, then again, they may perceive the carer, if female, to be their wife or girl-friend. The sexual behaviour produced by the client is in relation to the affection remembered for that person. Gently and tactfully try to distract the client away from the behaviour. If you act in an alarmed or angry way this will increase the client's distress. They will unconsciously know you are offended but not know why. With both confused or dementing clients the aim is to attempt to *help the client maintain their optimum level of functioning.*

How to focus the confused client

Ensure that reality orientation is used when maintaining a relationship with the client. Reinforce who you are and your function. Re-orientate the client to their environment. Provide a structured, certain routine. Focus on the client's strengths and abilities. Let them help you set the table for lunch or water the plants. Do not disempower the client. Engage the client in cognitive stimulation such as using games, painting, conversation and past memory material, for example, photographs and music. Do not let the client get tired.

Try to minimize disruptive behaviours in the client and make minimal demands on them for compliant behaviour. If the demands you make are too great this will increase the client's stress.

Try to ensure a safe environment. Low furniture like footstools can cause a client to fall over. Examine the client's environment for any hazard that will harm their wellbeing and safety. Ensure doors are clearly marked and large-faced clocks are used to tell the time. Social interaction and reality orientation groups can be helped by using newspapers, radio and television. These can help clients to be involved and relieve the symptoms of both confusion and dementia.

Your mental health

Activity 3.7   ■

Write down a short list of people you could turn to when you have problems and are not coping well.

■ ■

Looking after someone with confusion is a difficult and demanding job. Do not try to struggle on alone. Social workers, psychologists and nurses who have specialized in this area of care are a good source of help and advice. The Alzheimer's Disease Society provide excellent printed material and carers' support groups can also offer information. Your mental health is important (see Chapter 13).

Finally, remember to keep an accurate record of all your care given to a client. Record any untoward incident that may occur such as a fall or knock that happens to a client and ensure an incident form is filled in and your manager and the client's relatives are informed about the episode. Be honest in your dealings with relatives. Older people who are frail and vulnerable may occasionally fall and often bruise very badly as a result of the fall. Documenting and reporting the incident is part of good caring practice. Keeping relatives informed is essential, since unexplained bruises on a client may cause relatives to fear physical abuse. This concern is perfectly understandable. If the client's partner or relatives are involved in the care programme, any untoward incident is usually sympathetically understood.

Summary

Growing older should be a positive experience and yet most individuals are unprepared. For this to change the later years of life have to be viewed as meaningful and worthwhile. A personal ethic needs to be introduced while that person is still young, so that they can prepare for the third age. Most older people are very active and involved in the third age and it is this large group of older, active people who should be given a higher profile. A more positive view of the human life-span will contribute much to combat alienation and estrangement felt by the young in society. It is they who are often informed, insultingly, that the old are a burden. Is it then any wonder that young people are unable to prepare a personal ethic for their third age?

References

Caroline, H.A. (1993) Explorations of close friendship: a concept analysis, *Archives of Psychiatric Nursing*, August, **7** (4), 236.

Cowan, L. (1995) Positive images of ageing. *Elderly Care*, Jan/Feb, **7** (1), 14.

Forbes, S.B. (1994) Hope: an essential human need in the elderly. *Journal of Gerontological Nursing*, June, 5.

Garret, G. (1991) Relationships in later life. *Professional Nurse*, October **7** (6), 34.

Gross, R.D. (1987) *Psychology: The Science of Mind and Behaviour.* Edward Arnold, London.

Jaques, A. (1995) Psychiatry of old age, in *Companion to Psychiatric Studies.* R.E. Kendell & A.K. Zealley (eds), Churchill Livingstone, London.

Masters, W.H. & Johnson, V.E. (1966) *Human Sexual Response.* Littlebrown and Co. New York.

Mathieson, V., Sivertsen, L., Foreman, M.D. & Cronin-Stubbs, D. (1994) Acute confusion: nursing intervention in older patients. *Orthopaedic Nursing*, March/April, **13** (2), 21.

Miller, M.P. (1991) Factors promoting wellness in the aged person: an ethnographic study. *Advances in Nursing Science*, June, **13** (4), 38.

Scrutton, S. (1989) *Counselling for Older People: A Creative Response to Ageing.* Edward Arnold, London.

Shephard, R. (1990) The scientific basis of exercise prescribing for the very old. *American Geriatric Society*, JAGS (38), 62.

Further reading

Age Concern (1995) *HIV and AIDS and Older People, Medical Briefing.* Age Concern England, 1268 London Road, London SW16 4ER.

Alabaster, E. (1994) Architect of her own living. *Elderly Care*, May/June, **6** (3), 13.

Buckwalter, K. (1995) What successful approaches do you use in dealing with sexually aggressive patients/residents? *Journal of Gerontological Nursing*, September, **21** (9), 51.

Hadfield, N. (1994) Alzheimer's Disease, who cares? *Elderly Care*, March/April, **6** (2), 14.

Haigh, C. (1994) Gereontological gender gap. *Elderly Care*, Jan/Feb, **16** (1), 27.

Stuart, G.W. & Sundeen, S.J. (1995) *Principles and Practice of Psychiatric Nursing* Mosby, London.

Section 3
Promoting Independence

Chapter 4
Ethical Issues and the Older Person
David Carpenter

Overview

The first section of this chapter comprises an overview of ethics as a subject and a fundamental introduction to ethical theories, it aims to equip the reader with a basic set of analytical tools for effective analysis of substantive issues. The second section identifies major, general ethical issues associated with older people.

The final part of the chapter is divided into three further sections, each focusing on an a broad ethical issue. The first of these sections, 'Whose Risk is it Anyway?' addresses the problems associated with conflict between carers' desires to maximize clients' freedoms and choices and their duties to minimize risks.

The second section *Whose (Quality of) Life is is Anyway?* addresses issues concerned with exercising choices regarding treatment and care including life or death decisions.

The final section *Whose Business is it Anyway?* addresses the issue of confidentiality and its relationship to the duty to respect people.

Overall, the structure of the chapter allows the reader to gain a basic understanding of theory, apply that theory in identifying ethical issues associated with older people, and consolidate the learning by analysing more specific examples.

Key words

Ethics, facts, values, ought, deontology, consequentialism, utilitarianism, principles, beneficence, non-maleficence, justice, autonomy, confidentiality, euthanasia, paternalism, choices, electronic tagging.

Confronting the issues

'If I get old, infirm and dependent, I just want to be quietly put down.'

This is probably one of the most commonly stated views of young people contemplating old age. It is worth noting however, that the frequency of such statements tends to decline with advancing years; what seemed wise at 30 becomes a grim and frightening prospect at 60. Euthanasia is an obvious example of an ethical issue, but what exactly makes it an ethical issue, and why should we see it as pertinent to older people? You are probably not surprised to see an immediate focus on euthanasia, but is the author behaving ethically in establishing this early focus?

Any study of ethical issues and older people entails some investigation of the nature of ethics and individual perceptions of ethics and ethical issues.

Activity 4.1 ■

What ethical issues do you expect to be covered in this chapter? What is it that each of these issues has in common?

■ ■

What does your list say about you?

Ethical perceptions

Your list of ethical issues probably includes examples such as:

■ Confidentiality
■ Rights
■ Truth-telling
■ Euthanasia

You may also have included some topical issues such as electronic tagging and advance directives, the most common example of which is a living will. Interestingly, none of these issues are specifically and exclusively concerned with older people and their care. They all have some relevance, but equally, they are relevant to other care specialisms. In some ways this observation should be a source of relief. If ethical issues associated with caring for older people were argued to be special and unique it would invite accusations of discrimination and stereotyping. In short, a list of special ethical issues associated with caring for older people may, in itself, be unethical.

What makes an issue ethical?

What did you suggest that each of your issues had in common? You may have thought that they were each concerned with individual values or beliefs or that they were all concerned with the rightness or wrongness of human conduct. Ethics is concerned with what *ought* to be the case as opposed to some other subjects which are concerned with what *is* the case. For example, many people believe that the death penalty would act as a strong deterrent and that it should therefore be reinstated. Imagine that it was possible to undertake research and that there was irrefutable evidence that reinstatement of the death penalty would eliminate most murders. We could state that it *is* the case or it is a fact that reinstatement will eliminate most murders. The question of whether we *ought* to reinstate the death penalty is, however, a different question. Even if murder could be nearly eliminated we might still ask whether we *ought* to reinstate the death penalty.

True or false?

In your work as a health care worker you are constantly asking questions (sometimes only to yourself) and making statements. The answers to your questions may be true or false; your statements may equally be true or false. For example, you may ask what the normal body temperature is, or you may state that ampicillin is an antibiotic; your statement is true and you may or may not be given a true answer to your question. The truths of statements and the answers to questions can usually be established by investigation and gathering evidence.

Activity 4.2 ■

What is the difference between the following two statements?

(a) 'You are reading Chapter 4 on ethical issues'
(b) 'You ought to read Chapter 4 on ethical issues'

■ ■

Statement (a) is true, it is a fact, however it is not so easy to decide whether (b) is true or false or indeed, whether it even makes sense to suggest that it is a factual issue. Evidence of the truth of (a) is clear, yet would it even be possible to find evidence either in support of or against (b)? You may protest, you may argue that it is certainly true that you ought to read this chapter because it is concerned with ethical issues and they are important. Your protest is easily countered; even if ethical issues are important it will not follow that you should therefore read the chapter. Notice the similarity to the previous example, from the fact that capital punishment *would* act as a deterrent, it does not follow that it *should* be reinstated. We are, in effect, considering the relationship between a fact and a value, making the clear observation that facts cannot, in themselves, dictate values.

It is probably helpful to summarize at this point that ethical issues can be recognized because usually it is difficult, if not impossible, to state whether they are true or false.

What *ought* I to do?

Statements of fact can be tested by gathering evidence whereas ethical statements and questions tend to remain unanswered no matter how much factual evidence is gathered.

Activity 4.3 ■

 Can you recognize an ethical issue? Think about the last time you were at work, how many times did you ask yourself 'what ought I to do?' Try and recall an example of a situation prompting such a question.

■ ■

Your example will be personal, you may wish to consider the following case study and draw comparisons with your own situation.

Case study 1

 John's wife died some years ago, however, as a result of the dementing illness he suffers, John believes that his wife is alive and asks to see her almost every day. John is easily distracted and he can be reassured by simply saying that his wife will come tomorrow. Should you lie or should you tell John that his wife is dead?

The case example leaves you with a clear ethical question; 'what ought I to do?' It is tempting to try and answer this question like a factual one. You may keep looking for evidence in a vain attempt to answer the question.

Activity 4.4 ■

 Try listing all the factual questions you might ask.

■ ■

Your list may include questions such as:

■ The length of time since the death of John's wife
■ The severity of John's illness
■ Its rate of progress

Notice however, no matter what the answers to your questions might be, your original question remains *What ought I to do? Ought I to tell John that his wife is dead?*

You should now be able to recognize an ethical question and notice that it cannot be answered in the same way as a factual question. So how can we deal with an ethical question?

Activity 4.5 ■

 Before considering how to answer ethical questions it is worth noting just how many appear in your day to day work, and, more importantly, that most of the questions are not concerned with highly emotive issues, such as euthanasia. List as many situations as you can remember which have resulted in you asking 'What ought I to do?'

■ ■

Ethical analysis

Earlier it was suggested that ethics is concerned with analysis of what *ought* to be the case. What form might this analysis take? Ethical analysis is a matter of considering an issue in the light of an ethical theory. An ethical theory aims to explain why, for example, we should do A rather than B or why X is wrong. Ethical theories, like any other theories, do not tell us facts, but they can help explain or possibly defend our actions.

Activity 4.6   ■

Reflect back on Case study 1. What was your decision? If you decided to tell John that his wife was dead, what were the reasons for your choice? If you decided to distract John and lie, why did you choose to do so?

■ ■

You may have decided to tell John the truth because it is wrong to lie. You may feel that carers have a duty to tell their clients the truth. In reaching your decision you have employed a theory. Your theory may be summarized as: we ought to do our duty and our duty amounts to a set of rules including one which requires us to tell the truth.

On the other hand, you may have decided to lie to John because you thought that telling him the truth would cause him unnecessary distress. Again, in reaching your decision you have employed a theory. Your theory may be summarized as: we ought to think of the consequences of our actions and aim to maximize happiness or, at least, minimize misery.

Different view of ethics

Duty and consequence

The theoretical stance demonstrated in the former response is referred to as *deontological* whereas the latter response is that of a *consequentialist*. A deontologist argues that there are certain ethical duties which are good in themselves and should be obeyed regardless of any outcome. Stated rather simplistically this means, 'do as you would be done by', because we will all be subject to the same moral rules. A consequentialist argues that the morality of an action is measured by its outcome. Stated rather simplistically, this means 'all's well that ends well'. The most well-known form of consequentialism is utilitarianism, the view that an action is right when it produces the greatest balance of pleasure over pain among all people it affects (Morton, 1996). The observant reader will note that the word 'morality' was used. What is the difference between 'moral' and 'ethical'? This question often provokes a somewhat nit-picking argument. 'Ethics' and 'moral philosophy' are synonymous terms, there is little practical benefit in differentiating 'ethical' and 'moral'.

Subjectivism

You should notice that whether or not you lie to John, the decision can be defended on moral grounds using moral theory; the decision is not just a matter of personal choice. This is an important observation, many people argue that ethics is all rather subjective, in other words, whether an action is right or wrong, or whether one ought to do X rather than Y is just a matter of personal taste. This position is referred to as *subjectivism*, in some ways it is obvious that it is flawed. Whether or not one *ought* to tell John the truth is distinct from whether or not *I believe that* John ought to be told the truth.

Activity 4.7 ■■■■■■■■■■■■■■■■■■■■■■■■■■■■

The aim of this activity is to give you an opportunity to consolidate some of your learning. Consider the example of euthanasia and the more specific question of whether it ought to be available to older persons on request.
(a) How might a deontologist react to the question?
(b) How might a consequentialist react to the question?
(c) Is the ethics of euthanasia a subjective matter?

■■■■■■■■■■■■■■■■■■■■■■■■■■■■■■■■■■

Utilitarianism

You have probably suggested that a *deontologist* might argue that euthanasia is unethical since we have a duty not to kill. A *utilitarian* might support euthanasia if it resulted in maximizing pleasure or minimizing pain but they would nevertheless require safeguards to be established. For example, euthanasia would not be a good thing if it were to be performed involuntarily, since that would result in a greater balance of pain over pleasure. Imagine living in a society where you may, on the one hand, be reassured that you would not die in pain and with loss of dignity but on the other hand you may be killed for no better reason than you had reached the prescribed age. Euthanasia of this type could not be defended by either a deontologist or a utilitarian.

Right or wrong?

Is the rightness of euthanasia subjective? This question is more difficult to answer. If the matter is subjective then 'euthanasia is wrong' is equivalent to 'I believe that euthanasia is wrong'. It might readily be agreed that the rightness or wrongness of euthanasia is one thing, an individual's personal belief is a quite separate issue. In short, euthanasia is right or wrong independent of any individual's belief.

It is worth noting that deontologists and utilitarians do not necessarily arrive at different decisions. They may arrive at the same conclusions but for different reasons. The deontologist will uphold a rule that we should not kill a human being, a utilitarian will usually hold the same view because killing does not usually result in the maximization of pleasure and the minimization of pain.

Principlism

Deontology and consequentialism are, perhaps, best described as classical theories of ethics; they are interesting and can be used to analyse many day to day ethical issues. Both theories, however, have their critics and neither are particularly user friendly. A modern and increasingly popular approach to ethical analysis is *principlism*. Principlism holds that ethical issues and questions can be analysed with reference to clear and, arguably, uncontentious ethical principles. Each principle is accepted to be intrinsically good. In other words, it is fundamentally good rather than good because it results in a greater good such as a higher order duty or maximization of pleasure. In short, a principle does not stand in need of further ethical justification. Key exponents of principlism include Gillon (1984) and Beauchamp & Childress (1989).

Different principles

Different theorists propose different principles however the most frequently stated are:

- *Beneficence*: doing good for clients
- *Non-Maleficence*: avoiding harming clients
- *Justice*: treating clients fairly by properly allocating resources and respecting their rights
- *Respect for autonomy*: ensuring that clients' choices are respected

Activity 4.8   ■

 Reconsider Case study 1 and analyse it in the light of the principles.

■ ■

Usually the principle of beneficence requires us to tell the truth, however, in John's case, we could argue that it is not clear whether any good would result from telling him that his wife had died. We may conclude that telling John the truth would harm him, in which case doing so would be to disregard the principle of non-maleficence. While we may agree that John has a right to be told the truth we may also agree that he has a right not to experience what is, in effect, a daily bereavement. There is little doubt that under normal circumstances, telling a lie is an infringement of autonomy since exercising choice depends on accurate information being given. John, as a result of his dementing illness, has suffered a considerable impairment of autononmy; he has lost most of his former capacity to take decisions for himself. It is likely that John will be able to exercise some limited choices; for example, those regarding food or clothing. It is also likely that the distress resulting from a daily experience of bereavement will reduce his already limited capacity to make choices. On balance it could be argued, somewhat paradoxically, that John's autonomy may best be respected by lying to him.

It should now be clear that ethical issues can be analysed using ethical theories; such analyses do not yield answers which are either true or false. An ethical analysis may constitute an explanation of one's actions or, more strongly, in some situations it may act as a defence.

It should be noted that an honest analysis may well conflict with one's personal beliefs or wishes. You may for example, have decided that you *ought* not tell John the truth but you have a personal inclination to do so. If you act on the basis of your analysis you can always explain your actions, if however, you act on the basis of personal desires, there may be no defensible explanation to offer. This may mean that the oft quoted maxim 'always let your conscience be your guide' is not as sound as most people think.

Now that we have investigated the nature of ethics as a subject and the elements of ethical theory, it is possible to explore some key issues.

What are the main issues?

At the beginning of this chapter we assembled a list of ethical issues to establish what they had in common.

We noted that there were probably no ethical issues uniquely pertaining to older persons and suggested that there was something worrying about the tendency to raise euthanasia as an immediate example of an ethical issue concerned with the care of older people! Particular problems associated with old age do, however, raise particular, if not unique, ethical issues. Most of these problems relate to autonomy. Remember that autonomy is the capacity to choose for oneself and the principle of autonomy requires carers to respect clients' choices.

Activity 4.9 ■■■■■■■■■■■■■■■■■■■■■■■■■■■■■■

What do you think these autonomy related problems are?

■■■■■■■■■■■■■■■■■■■■■■■■■■■■■■■■■■

Autonomy related issues

We have already encountered one autonomy related example, that of impairment resulting from dementing illness. The concept of autonomy includes acting for oneself as well as thinking for oneself. Physical infirmity may well compromise a person's ability to act, at least with a degree of safety, for him or herself. Is it ethical to let an older person live alone according to his wishes even if serious risks are present? Very serious illness may result in a loss of autonomy or, at least, a complete inability to exercise autonomy. If a person has a serious cerebro-vascular accident (stroke) he or she may be left unconscious and will not be able to make their choices known directly. We may agree that we should continue to respect this person's autonomy but establishing the choices he or she would have made can prove difficult. Other specific examples of autonomy related ethical issues can be summarized as resulting from varying degrees of impairment of autonomy of thought and action.

Autonomy is not the only ethical principle; most of the problems we encounter will require analysis from the perspectives of most, if not all of the principles.

Some principles to consider

Given the foregoing discussion it is now possible to describe some of the most frequently encountered issues in terms of principles. The following principles are not intended to be all-inclusive and, again, it must be remembered that the issues stated are not only associated with older people.

First, there is frequently a conflict between encouraging or permitting maximum independence and a risk of harm. Most older people wish to lead independent lives in their own homes but illness or increasing frailty can result in serious risks, for example, risks of falling or suffering hypothermia or remaining undiscovered following a serious acute illness. Is it ethical to allow such risks? Is it ethical *not* to allow older people to take such risks?

Secondly, advances in health care have resulted in what seems to be an ever increasing range of life-saving and life-prolonging interventions. These advances are often seen as a 'mixed blessing'. On the one hand there is the relief of knowing that a worthwhile life can be saved, on the other hand there is the fear that a life of pain and misery could be prolonged. Although these advances are beneficial, there is still the worry that not enough resources are available to sustain them, thus raising a question of justice and allocation of the limited resources.

Finally, in many cases, advancing age means increasing dependence upon others. The inevitable result of such dependence is some erosion of privacy, it is simply not possible to keep oneself to oneself. If invasions of privacy are managed with care there need not be any adverse effect upon the dignity of a person. Similarly, if carers work with integrity, confidences of older people will be respected. There is always the danger however that dependence will result in assaults upon dignity and careless breaches of confidence. Furthermore, dependence can result in people being seen as problems. Loss of personhood and a new identity as a 'problem' raises some of the most worrying ethical issues. All people deserve respect and care. Problems merely need management and solutions.

Activity 4.10 ■

 Try and summarize each of the issues discussed using ethical theory or ethical principles.

■ ■

Analysing the principles by using ethics

The first issue raises the problem of respecting autonomoy but increasing risk as result of doing so. The principles of beneficence and non-malefi-cence can lead us to be over-protective, taking away an older person's limited independence for his or her own good. This tendency is called paternalism, basically a well-intended intervention aimed to be in the best interests of the older person, but nevertheless not desired by that person. It is also noteworthy that an unwanted intervention represents an inap-propriate use of resources and is therefore unjust.

The second issue has much in common with the first, but the specific examples are more worrying given their life or death focus. You may ask whether it is beneficent to give life-saving or life-prolonging treatment to a person who does not want it. While it may be easy to see how we can respect the autonomy of an older person who has the capacity to refuse or consent to treatment, what about the person who has lost the capacity to make decisions, but has left instructions, perhaps in the form of a living will? Living wills will be discussed in more detail later.

The isssue is not only about letting people die as a result of treatment refusal, a passive form of euthanasia, it could equally be about a person requesting life-prolonging treatment in circumstances where health pro-fessionals may regard such an intervention as futile. Many health profes-sionals believe, with some justification, that some treatment does more harm than good; in other words a balance between beneficence and non-maleficence cannot be achieved. While the professionals' views may be perfectly valid, it is still possible that a client may wish to commence or continue with treatment which does little more than prolong a life of pain and suffering. Maybe the lesson here is that goodness or benefit is in the 'eye of the beholder'. An intervention may be beneficent *because* it is wanted (respects autonomy) rather than for any objective outcome.

The third example should just serve as a reminder that respect for all persons could be seen as an ultimate ethical goal. When a person is reduced to a 'problem' it could be agreed that we have lost all sense of morality since one of its primary objectives, the interests of the individual, has been lost. Respecting confidences is often seen by health professionals as intrinsically good, in other words, good in itself; this is a mistake. Respecting confidences helps to maintain privacy which, in turn, is essential to personal identity. An indiscrete communication of confidential information is an obvious assault on the person.

Now that we have considered some ethical theory and identified some ethical issues we will consider some substantive examples.

Whose risk is it anyway?

Health care workers sometimes feel that they cannot win! On the one hand they are encouraged to ensure that older people enjoy as much freedom as possible and the use of any restraint including locked doors, and chairs which are difficult to vacate, is frowned upon. On the other hand, paid carers working in the private or public sectors are conscious of the threat of litigation; 'let this person wander freely but if he comes to harm we will sue you!' How can the carer win? The carer cannot win, but why should he or she anyway? It is the client that needs to win not the carer!

In a way, the dilemma outlined above is artificial; it results from the creation of two contradictory rules both of which, we believe, must be respected.

- *Rule 1* Allow maximum freedom and thereby maximum opportunities to come to harm.
- *Rule 2* Minimize opportunities for coming to harm therefore restrict freedoms.

As suggested earlier, this dilemma may be artificial. Applying rules to people in this way may not be a good idea. When faced with a question of how much freedom to allow, it may be better to analyse the particular situation rather than apply any arbitrary rule.

Activity 4.11 ■

 Imagine yourself as an older person, how would you wish to be treated? Would you wish to be subject to rule 1 or would you prefer rule 2? Do you know another person who would wish to be treated the opposite way to you?

■ ■

Freedom of choice

It is likely that you have concluded that some people like to 'live dangerously' while others prefer to 'play it safe' and neither would wish to be subjected to an arbitrary rule, particularly if it contrasts with their normal attitude to life.

The moral of the story is to think before instituting general rules, which may include the much-loved policies so many institutions find it necessary to create. In some ways this problem is an example of trying to address an ethical question as though it were a factual one. The major ethical issue is respect for autonomy, which may require treating people on an individual basis which, after all, is commended as good practice anyway. Just as we may baulk at the idea of giving every client the same outfit of clothing, we should equally baulk at giving every client the same degree of freedom.

Helping a client to choose

One way of dealing with our dilemma would be to simply respect the desires of the client. If the client wishes to enjoy maximum freedom, it is not good to impose restrictions. Equally, if a client does not wish to take any risks, including, for example, a short walk, it is not good to impose it. Some carers will feel disinclined to allow maximum freedom on the basis of the risk being too high, but it should be clear that the risks are the client's and taking risks are an inevitable consequence of his or her freedom. On the issue of litigation, it should be obvious that a carer cannot be sued for not restricting the liberty of a client who wishes to enjoy it. Indeed, the reverse could well be true.

Making choices for the client

A simple solution requiring us to always respect the client's wishes may not always be available. What should we do if a client is confused or expresses desires we know to be uncharacteristic? Should we allow clients to do as they wish, even though their behaviour may be entirely out of keeping? The big danger is the tendency to accept behaviour with which we are comfortable, while rejecting behaviour we find inconvenient. It is not unusual to find a carer claiming that a particular client has 'chosen' not to shave, to look untidy, to wear mismatching clothes. Did the client really choose or was it simply convenient to claim that he had chosen and, moreover, to claim that any attempt to change him would constitute a serious infringement of his liberty! It is possible that the client had made a choice; it is equally possible that the carer had a convenient excuse for not intervening, and moreover, an apparently ethical defence. The matter is relatively easily settled by establishing whether the client had the capacity to choose. Inconsistency is remarkably common, we have clients 'choosing' to look a mess. There are also, apparently, clients 'choosing' to give up smoking or 'choosing' to retire to bed at a ridiculously early hour. Isn't it strange how clients always seem to 'choose' that which coincides with the interests of their carers!

When the capacity to choose is no longer evident, carers may have to choose on behalf of clients. One way of making such choices defensibly is to make the choice you sincerely believe the client would have made had he or she been able. Notice that this precludes general rules and, also, it may entail making decisions with which you may not necessarily agree.

Activity 4.12 ■

Consider the clients in your care, how many are subjected to rules to which it can reasonably be assumed they would object, if only they had the capacity to do so? Consider things like smoking, drinking alcohol, eating a so-called healthy diet, bed times...

Next time you help an older person get dressed, consider whether the style and colour of the clothing would have been their choice.

■ ■

If we return to our earlier focus on how much freedom we should allow, we can now agree that we should respect autonomy either by respecting choices of clients or, where clients do not have the capacity to choose, making choices for them on the basis of what we sincerely believe they would have done themselves.

Electronic tagging

Older people suffering from dementing illnesses frequently wander, one way of managing this is the introduction of electronic tagging, but is this ethical? It is tempting to make an immediate and resounding response of 'NO'. There is, however, scope to undertake a more considered analysis. Most forms of tagging that have been introduced are simple systems. An alarm is triggered as the tagged person attempts to pass through the doorway thus providing an opportunity to retrieve them from harm's way. There is little difference between this system and merely locking the door except, of course, the confused client is deceived into believing that he or she has complete freedom. Such a criticism may be unfair because such a system should not be applied indiscriminately. Only the most confused and most at risk need tagging. Such discrimination is desirable, however, we have already met the tendency to introduce arbitrary rules and to create policy. Equally, there is always the danger that a system designed to protect clients could ultimately be used to protect over-defensive health professionals, particularly in times of staffing crises.

Other kinds of tagging are rather more sophisticated, allowing constant awareness of a client's whereabouts while not imposing any immediate obstacles to freedom. In brief, the client can become a 'blip' on a screen and the screen covers a wide geographical area. This type of tagging allows maximum freedom while ensuring that no client is lost and at risk of such outcomes such as hypothermia. Tagging of this nature is clearly advantageous if the only other alternative is a significant restriction of movement, for example, remaining within an institutional setting.

Activity 4.13 ■

 What are your views on tagging? Take this opportunity to prepare a few arguments both in favour and against the practice.

■ ■

When to use tagging

You probably feel that it depends on the circumstances. Tagging can be beneficial if the only other alternative is a greater restriction of freedom. On the other hand, it would be best avoided if at all possible, most obviously where no restriction of freedom is necessary. If you recall the earlier discussion you may also have noted that the value of tagging will, to some extent depend on the nature of the client in question.

Some people enjoy wandering. How many people do you know who stroll aimlessly but pleasurably? Other people tend to be more purposeful, they only go out with a specific reason in mind and only walk to a specific destination. Imagine two people being seriously demented, a former wanderer and a former non-wanderer, in their demented states, both may be equally inclined to wander and both can present similar challenges to carers. Problems identified in the care plans of each of these clients may be identical, however, it may not only be defensible, but also ethically necessary to treat them very differently. We could tag the person who was previously inclined to wander and, if anything, encourage him or her on their way. On the other hand we may attempt to limit the wanderings of the formerly purposeful person. We will probably never be able to determine the actual wishes of either person, but we can at least make an assumption that each would have wished to maintain their previous way of life. We should never treat people similarly merely because they happen to pose similar problems.

Whose (quality of) life is it anyway?

Respecting choices in some situations can be a matter of life or death; obvious examples include withholding or withdrawing life-saving or life-prolonging treatment. The treatment in question need not be 'high tech', it can be a simple issue of a course of antibiotics or simple naso-gastric tube feeding. The anticipated effects of the treatment can range from an immediate saving of life to an addition of several years of life.

Treatment is another area where blind application of rules is not easily defended, particularly where those rules purport to be founded on some objective criterion. Such criteria are frequently ageist as evidenced in policies of witholding some forms of treatment merely because the client is of a certain age. It is equally problematic to suggest that all clients regardless of age should enjoy equal access to treatment. It is undeniable that with, advancing years, some treatment results in more harm than good, in which case age becomes a relevant criterion which can influence decisions.

There are many examples of situations where older persons have received treatment on the basis of having a so-called right to it and such a right being demanded by a well-meaning but nevertheless naive 'advocate'. Such treatment may result in no appreciable benefit and possibly significant harm. In brief, rules, again are problematic and can be summarized as follows.

(1) It is probably wrong not to treat a person merely because he or she is of a certain age.
(2) It is probably wrong to demand that an older person is treated merely because a younger person in similar circumstances would have received treatment.

Who should receive treatment?

How then should we decide who should receive what forms of treatment?

Stated somewhat simplistically, a defensible maxim could be, 'treat those who wish to be treated, do not treat those who do not wish to be treated.' We might add a caveat that the wish should be the product of deliberated thought based on sound information with no obvious coercive influence. This moral maxim is obviously related to the similar legal requirement to seek consent before proceeding with care and treatment. We should remember that it is a person's right to refuse treatment that is likely to save and prolong life, even if that treatment entails little or no discomfort. It is equally a person's right to accept treatment that may be painful and uncomfortable and only likely to result in some minimal extension of life. It is the health care workers in both situations described above who experience the greatest difficulties! While they may respond to either of the situations described with incredulity, ultimately it is possible to resolve conflict by adhering to the wishes of the client.

> 'I know that you could provide care and treatment which would save my life but I don't want it.'

> 'I know that I am dying but if you can give me treatment which might add a few extra moments to my life, I would like it.'

In some cases it is not so easy to establish the immediate wishes of the client. Consider the following case study.

Case study 2

Mrs Longman was attending a large public event when she collapsed following a cardiac arrest. Some nearby paramedics came immediately to her assistance and began resuscitation measures. Mrs Longman's son, who was accompanying her asked the paramedics to stop because his mother had always made it clear that in such circumstances she would not wish to be resuscitated. Mr Longman's protests were ignored, the resuscitation was continued to a successful conclusion and Mrs Longman was eventually admitted to hospital.

On admission, staff established that Mrs Longman had been a very active 70 year old with a strong interest in gardening and a busy life. Her cardiac arrest had been the result of a momentary arrythmia rather than serious coronary artery disease and her prognosis was good. Mr Longman insisted that his mother should be noted as 'not for resuscitation' and she confirmed the instruction when she fully regained her senses.

Activity 4.14 ■

What are your views on this case? Try and reflect upon your reaction to Mrs Longman and her son.

■ ■

It is likely that you are as shocked as the staff were in this case. Why should a woman who has been restored to health still wish to be left to die? You may not just be suprised, you may equally be indignant! How ungrateful can clients get!

Life or death decisions

When a nurse took the trouble to sit and talk to Mrs Longman and ask her to explain her decision, everything became clear.

Mrs Longman explained that she had indeed been healthy up to the time of her cardiac arrest and she was quite sure that that was the best time to die. Mrs Longman felt that she had been deprived of a peaceful, dignified, pain-free death occurring on a pleasant afternoon while she was out with her son. She saw the future as holding the possibility of increasing disability, frailty, disease, pain and discomfort. Why should any person desire to end life in such circumstances?

Perhaps the simple moral of this story is that the interventions of health professionals are rarely good in themselves. They are only good when they are desired by clients. Mrs Longman's treatment was not good; she did not want it. It is equally possible, however, that another person who may be dying and experiencing pain and discomfort may nevertheless wish to be resuscitated in the event of a cardiac arrest. Treatment, which may achieve little more than a prolongation of pain and suffering, can be good if it is wanted.

To summarize: treatment and care should be *offered* to clients who can *choose* to accept or refuse it. The assumption that treatment is good in itself and should therefore be given regardless of the client's wishes is an obvious example of paternalism; the view that we as carers, always know best. Decisions regarding whether treatment should be offered are frequently informed by assessments of quality of life and judgements about the anticipated effectiveness of the treatment. It would, of course, be quite wrong to ignore these factors. What is the point of giving treatment that will be ineffective? What is the point of giving treatment that will have a negative impact on the quality of life of the client?

These considerations alone are not enough, though, to make decisions. The client's own view is equally, if not more, important. Using the ethical theory we presented earlier we can say that beneficence is a goal for carers, but we should not lose sight of our duty to respect autonomy.

Rights and duties

Some health professionals misunderstand these basic principles; it is not unusual to hear claims of a right to treat clients. Health professionals have no more of a right to treat clients than a painter has to paint your house! Both have duties to perform their work to a reasonable standard when they have received instructions from the client.

Duties to treat people who wish to be treated are all well and good, but at the time of her cardiac arrest, Mrs Longman was in no position to express her wishes. We have already considered the case of the demented person who may not be able to express desires. Other people who may not be able to express their desires may be those who have suddenly become confused or unconscious, perhaps as a result of an accident or an acute medical crisis. It would be quite wrong to suggest that the desires of people in such situations do not exist, it is simply not possible to *express* them. Many people fear the prospect of being in a state whereby they are unable to express their own views, yet life or death decisions must be made. This fear could be alleviated if we could make provision for such an eventuality in the form of an advance directive.

Living wills

An advance directive is a decision concerning possible future medical care and treatment made by a competent client in anticipation of a future loss of competence. Such a decision can be stated in the form of a *living will*, a practice which has been the subject of much debate. The ethical value of a living will is that it allows autonomy to be respected even after a client has reached a point where he is no longer able to exercise it; legally such a client is referred to as 'incompetent'.

Living wills frequently state a client's refusal of future, potentially life-saving, or life-prolonging treatment, however, they may equally state a client's wish to receive such treatment. It is therefore quite wrong to see living wills as a form of suicide or passive euthanasia, which is a death brought about intentionally by witholding or withdrawing life-saving or life-prolonging treatment.

The major debates surrounding living wills are both ethical and legal. The advantages of living wills from an ethical point of view are clear, but there are equally dangers. One danger is the possibility of an older person being coerced into 'signing away' future treatment rights; coercion might emanate from unscrupulous relatives or result from political and social pressure. This is an obvious danger, however, it does not constitute a valid argument against living wills, rather, it constitutes a worry about their potential abuse. This is not a sufficient reason to reject a proposition however, it is a good reason for regulating it with caution. A good example of a well deliberated analysis of the issue can be found in the report of Age Concern and the Centre of Medical Law and Ethics working party (1988).

Living wills can make future desires clear in that they allow consent to and refusal of treatment which could be deemed to be medically beneficial. They cannot be used to demand treatment which is not medically indicated, nor can they be used to demand an intervention which would constitute a crime, including active euthanasia or 'mercy killing'. It must be stated, unequivocally, that the intentional killing of a client, even at his request, is unlawful. Legally the issue may be clear, though perhaps, a little two-faced. It is lawful to administer pain-relieving drugs at potentially fatal dosages so long as the primary intention is to relieve pain rather than kill. According to Kennedy & Grubb (1994), the law regarding mercy killing is unlikely to change and 'the doctor faced with a patient *in extremis* and asking to die will have to resort to the "double speak" of purporting to relieve pain while bringing about death, making sure that the agent bringing about death is one recognised by other doctors as a pain reliever' (Kennedy & Grubb, 1994).

It is not possible, in the confines of this short chapter, to analyse arguments for and against euthanasia in any depth. However, it would be wrong to conclude this section without considering at least some of the arguments.

Activity 4.15 ■■■■■■■■■■■■■■■■■■■■■■■■■■■

 What arguments, both for and against euthanasia, are you most familiar with. Take a few moments to consider them.

■■■■■■■■■■■■■■■■■■■■■■■■■■■■■■

Euthanasia

The most commonly stated argument is the one that involves drawing an analogy between human beings and other animals. Proposers of euthanasia argue that we consider it not only humane but a positive duty to relieve other animals of their suffering yet we do not extend a similar consideration to human beings. They rarely state the conclusion of the argument explicitly because it exposes the flaw.

The conclusion can be stated thus: as we are all animals we should be treated in a similar way. Most people would not wish to be treated in the same way as their dogs, or for that matter, their goldfish, merely because they are all animals! Human beings are different to other animals, the precise nature of those differences, including their ethical relevance, is a matter of debate but the fact that they are different is not in question. Given that there are differences between human beings and other animals, there are no grounds for arguing that they should be treated similarly unless, of course, the differences are not ethically relevant. The ethical relevance of the differences between human beings is a matter of complex debate which cannot be addressed here, however, we can conclude that the 'simple' argument supported by so many people, is not so simple after all.

Most people agree that there are conceivable situations in which a person could experience extremes of unremitting pain, such that the only possible 'solution' is euthanasia. Moreover, the suggestion, in this case, is that euthanasia is not only ethically acceptable, it is ethically demanded. It is relatively easy to construct case examples where euthanasia is apparently ethical. The main argument against the introduction of a law permitting euthanasia is the potential for abuse. Again, it should be emphasized that the fact that euthanasia may be abused does not constitute a valid argument against its introduction. We can summarize by recognizing that there are arguments both for and against euthanasia; however, in this country it remains unlawful.

Whose business is it anyway?

Earlier in the chapter it was argued that a breach of confidence could be seen as a violation of a person's autonomy. This is perhaps, an unfamiliar way of describing the issue. You are probably aware that you have a duty not to disclose confidential information but you may not have ever considered precisely why.

Activity 4.16 ■

  Why should carers offer confidentiality? Try to list some reasons.

■ ■

Confidentiality

You may have found the activity quite difficult; this is because confidentiality is probably not, in itself, of any value. Of course a promise of confidentiality is, in itself, ethically important, because promises should be kept. Confidentiality in health care contexts is an instrumental good. In other words, while not a good in itself, it can lead to good. If we offer a confidential service to clients, they will share information freely, this information may be vital in determining the best possible care and treatment. It is obvious that the client is the ultimate beneficiary of a confidential service. Conversely, if confidences are breached, clients would be disinclined to share sensitive information and it would be difficult, if not impossible, to provide appropriate care and treatment. It is worth noting that this latter point is a strong example of a utilitarian argument; good is maximized by not breaching confidences.

Breaching confidentiality

It is also possible to develop a deontologically based argument in support of respecting confidences; giving away information about other people removes an important choice and therefore disregards autonomy. Deontologists would argue that we have a duty to respect autonomy and that that duty would normally require us to respect confidentiality. The term 'normally' in this context is important, there are situations where confidentiality can defensibly be breached; most health professionals are aware of these situations and an intentional breach of confidence is always a matter of considered professional judgement. Intentional breaches of confidence usually take place with the client's knowledge, if not consent. Unintentional breaches may only become known to the client after the event and may be the source of great distress.

Do you tell the relatives?

Many carers are aware of the dangers of divulging confidential information to bodies such as the press though, of course, it is rare that the press shows much interest in older people in the care of others; most interest is shown by relatives and friends.

Many carers forget that disclosing confidential information to a client's relatives is nevertheless unethical; ironically, it is not unusual for a client to show little concern about information disclosed to strangers while being horrified at the prospect of that same information being disclosed to a relative.

It is noteworthy that, all too often, carers share information with relatives of clients without giving the matter a second thought! Despite popular belief to the contrary, relatives do not have any right to confidential information. Carers should always, as a matter of course, establish which members of a client's family should be informed of his or her progress by asking the client. Having established a line of communication, carers should still seek consent from the client before passing on information.

Summary

This chapter has explained ethical theories and discussed various issues associated with older people.

In conclusion it is worth reiterating the relationship between respecting confidences and recognizing every client as a unique individual whose privacy and dignity should always be respected.

References

Age Concern/Centre of Medical Law and Ethics (1988) *Report* Arnold, London.

Beauchamp, T.L. & Childress, J.F. (1989) *Principles of Biomedical Ethics*, 3rd edn. O.U.P. Oxford.

Gillon R. (1986) *Philosophical Medical Ethics*. Wiley, Chichester.

Kennedy I. & Grubb A. (1994) *Medical Law: Text with Materials*. Butterworths, London.

Morton, A. (1996) *Philosophy in Practice: An Introduction to the Main Questions*. Blackwell, Oxford.

Further reading

Hadden, B. (1994) *The Ageing Parent Handbook*. Thorsons, an Imprint of Harper Collins Publishers, London.

Wilcock, G.K. & Muir Gray, J.A. (1981) *Our Elders*. Oxford University Press, Oxford.

Chapter 5
Advocacy
Ruth Ashworth

Overview

By introducing the concept of advocacy, it is the aim of this chapter to:

■ Stimulate the reader into how to value clients' opinions and views
■ Consider how these can be put into everyday practice
■ Value the individual and empower him or her to make an informed choice
■ Consider good practice including respecting the privacy and dignity of the client

Key words

Accountability, advocacy, attitudes, beliefs, communication, confidentiality, decision-making, dignity, empowerment, equality, equal opportunities, informed choice, multi-disciplinary approach, negotiation, opinion, values, working in partnership.

Definition of advocacy

The word 'advocacy' stems from the Latin verb *advocare* which means to summon, to call for help or to advise. In Roman times this verb had strong legal connections and connotations. *The Oxford Dictionary of Current English* (1989) defines the word advocate as being 'one who supports or speaks in favour of, one who pleads for another.'

At the end of the twentieth century advocacy can be observed to be at work in many different areas, for example animal welfare, conservation and environment, racial awareness, and political prisoners.

Campaigning on behalf of others

Activity 5.1 ■■■■■■■■■■■■■■■■■■■■■■■■■■■■■■

 Think of five different areas which are examples of people campaigning on behalf of others.

■■■■■■■■■■■■■■■■■■■■■■■■■■■■■■■■■■

In the caring profession the term advocacy is still under debate. How far the role extends in its formal sense is not fully clear and therefore is open to interpretation. Below are some descriptions of advocacy, or the activity ascribed to it:

■ 'Assisting the patient by making such representations as he would make himself if he were able' (UKCC, 1989).
■ 'Ensuring that no one usurps the needs, rights, and humanity of patients' (Wells, 1988) to lend the patient strength.
■ Such empowering may assist the patient or the client to 'Endure and if possible to avoid a situation so desperate he would be pushed beyond his endurance' (Copp, 1986).
■ 'Involves assuming some responsibilities for another person who for one reason or another is unable to manage the situation effectively for himself' (Carpenter, 1992).
■ 'Informing the patient of his rights in a particular situation, making sure that he has all the necessary information to make an informed decision, supporting him in the decision he makes, and protecting and safeguarding his interests' (Clark, 1982).

Activity 5.2 ■■■■■■■■■■■■■■■■■■■■■■■■■■■■■■

(a) What is your initial reaction to the above definitions? Is there anything you particularly like? Is there anything you disagree with? An observation you may have made is that the client is referred to as being male where gender is mentioned. Is this significant at all?
(b) Which one is closest to your own understanding, and why?

■■■■■■■■■■■■■■■■■■■■■■■■■■■■■■■■■■■■■■

Advocacy in its formal sense

Advocacy can be interpreted in both a formal and informal way. When advocacy in care becomes involved in political activity, or within a legal framework, or action involving negotiation with management, this type of advocacy can cause controversy and conflict, often reflected in media coverage.

To illustrate this the United Kingdom Central Council Code of Professional Conduct (UKCC, 1994) for registered nurses imply that advocacy has a formal role to play. There are three clauses. They should:

(1) 'Report to an appropriate person or authority, having regard to the physical, psychological and social effects on patients and clients, any circumstances in the environment of care which could jeopardise standards of practice.' (No. 11)
(2) 'Report to an appropriate person or authority any circumstances in which safe and appropriate care for patients and clients cannot be provided.' (No 12)

(3) 'Report to an appropriate person or authority where it appears that the health or safety of colleagues is at risk, as such circumstances may compromise standards of practice and care.' (No. 13)

Although health care assistants are not bound by this code of conduct, these are helpful guidelines for practice. However, they are very broad and so open to interpretation. An important principle to remember when making decisions about action is that every individual worker whether they qualified or not are accountable for the care provided.

Some illustrations of advocacy in its formal sense might be where a worker reports to management unsafe practices, or where equipment is dangerous, or where clients are abused.

Activity 5.3 ■■■■■■■■■■■■■■■■■■■■■■■■■■■

Describe what action you would take, and why in these situations:

(a) You arrive on duty for a night shift. The person in charge seems stressed and smells very strongly of alcohol and on return from your break you find her asleep.

(b) One morning you are assisting Ivy, a 78 year old lady, to wash. She seems very upset and tells you that yesterday morning a carer stood on her toes and pulled her hair until she cried, and warned her that if she caused any trouble there would be worse to come. Ivy then tells you this is confidential and asks you not to tell anyone.

(c) For the last five weeks in the older people's home there have been staff shortages. In addition, this week one member of staff has started a day release training course of a year's duration and another is on indefinite sick leave. Although not qualified, you feel under pressure to take on more responsibility that you have not been trained for. Twice this week you have been left in charge.

■■■■■■■■■■■■■■■■■■■■■■■■■■■■■■■■■■

These situations will place you in a very difficult position and you will be forced to consider many questions such as:

In (a) Do I report the person? If not, why not?
        Do I remain silent for fear of causing trouble?
        Do I wake the person and enquire about their health?
        In whose best interest am I serving?
In (b) Do I report the person? If not, why not?
        Do I remain silent for fear of causing trouble?
        Do I break the patient's request for confidentiality? If so how would I cope with it?
        In whose best interest am I serving?
In (c) Should I continue to take on more responsibility?
        In whose best interest am I serving if I do?
        Am I putting patients at risk?

Advocacy in the informal sense

Advocacy in its everyday informal context can be a subtle quiet process between the carer and the client. It is about helping a client feel in control of a situation, empowering and supporting clients in their choices and decision making. Examples of this type of empowerment could be assisting a client choose what he or she would like to eat, or if and when they would like a wash or a bath. It is about ensuring a client is involved in choosing what happens to him or her and that the care provided is of good quality and tailored to that individual. Even small things like using a client's own soap or cleaning an electric razor between each use gives a message to clients and co-workers that the client is viewed as an individual and is the focus of care. Goodwin & Mangan (1985) question whether or not carers may have a higher standard for themselves than for clients:

> If it was necessary to use a patient's cup for yourself would you wash it out thoroughly? If so is it because you might catch dementia, or because you know the patient's cups are sometimes not clean? Would you make the same effort if it was for another patient's use, or do they have different standards of cleanliness? . . . if you were at the hairdressers and you noticed the brush she was about to use was full of other people's hair and dandruff, would you walk straight out? Or just sit there and chat away merrily?

Being vulnerable

Being in hospital or living in an older people's home (no matter how high the standard of care), or feeling ill or confused can have the result of a client being more vulnerable and less independent. This is why it is vitally important for the health care worker to make a special effort to work in partnership with the client to ensure that he or she is making an informed choice and is fully in agreement about the care given.

Rights and choices

Brown (1985) suggests there are four broad areas of needs or rights:

(1) The right to a good quality of care, which should be individual
(2) The right to equality in access to the care needed
(3) The right to be fully informed
(4) The right to know alternatives to the treatment offered

Activity 5.4 ■

Imagine you are staying in bed and breakfast accommodation. The toilet and bathroom are at the end of the corridor. Rate these in order of importance:

(a)   Being able to lock your bedroom door
(b)   Expecting people to knock on your door before entering your room
(c)   Being able to lock the toilet door
(d)   Being able to lock the bathroom door
(e)   Knowing that no-one has access to your belongings i.e. your purse/
        wallet, your bag/case and your drawers.

How did you make your choices?
Does your choice differ from your colleagues?
Is there a difference in what you could expect in privacy and choice
between staying in a hotel or a residential home, why?

■■■■■■■■■■■■■■■■■■■■■■■■■■■■■■■■■

Sometimes pressures stand in the way of health care workers which
make it difficult, or even prevent them creating an environment where
clients are able to participate in making choices for themselves.

Activity 5.5   ■■■■■■■■■■■■■■■■■■■■■■■■■■

 Think of an activity in the last week where you feel a client could have
been given more opportunity to choose for him or herself.

■■■■■■■■■■■■■■■■■■■■■■■■■■■■■■■■■

Your list may consist of:

■   Choosing from the menu
■   Deciding when to get up or go to bed
■   Wanting to use the telephone
■   Choosing a television or radio programme

What was it about this situation which prevented the client from having
more freedom to choose?
    You may have thought of:

■   Something unexpected happening in the environment
■   Being short of staff
■   Feeling under stress

Reflecting on this situation, can you think of any strategies you could use
in another similar situation if this occurs again? Looking back at a situation
and trying to see what was positive and negative about it can be a useful way
to examine and evaluate care given. This process is called reflective practice
and can be used as a process to look at and develop standards of care.

Negotiating decisions

Communication is the most effective way of finding out how a client views
his or her needs, providing information and discovering what the client's

choice is. Verbal and non-verbal communication are both equally important to take into consideration in the interpretation of a client's response and the delivery of care. Chapter 2 looks in depth at communicating effectively with clients.

Working in partnership

Working in partnership with clients is a vitally important concept to adopt in any therapeutic relationship. This means working closely with clients in a way which encourages clients to express themselves equally and have control over decisions without feeling they are being overpowered by health professionals. There are situations where clients are not fully able to express themselves and it is difficult to know what their choice would be. Involving the multi-disciplinary care team and the client's family and friends may be an appropriate source to draw upon in such circumstances.

It is useful to remember that it is no easier for clients to make decisions than it is for ourselves.

Activity 5.6 ■

Think of a time when you were faced with making an important decision, for example, moving house.
Who did you discuss the decision with?
What helped you make your mind up?
Now imagine you are in hospital and are unable to return home. You are faced with moving to an older people's home.
Describe your feelings.
What are your worries or concerns?
Do you feel you have any control or choice?
How do you express the above and who do you talk to?
Next, imagine you are faced with the same situation. However, this time you have had a cerebral-vascular accident or stroke and have lost the ability to speak and are unable to write. Describe the outcome, highlighting any differences.

■ ■

Situations and resources can have an impact on communication with the result that the provision of information and the facilitation of client choice may be less effective.

Activity 5.7 ■

You are visiting clients in the community on behalf of Babul Ahmed, a Bengali speaking associate nurse, who is on leave. The first visit is to Jamil Hussain, who needs his catheter bag and tubing changed and some assistance with a shower. Jamil's first language is Bengali, he appears to know a few words of English and gives the impression of understanding quite a few more words. Husnara Begum, his granddaughter, aged 11 years, is off from school and offers to translate for you. You have four more visits to do following this one.

From the following list select which action most closely resembles your own:

(a)   You do the care required without involving Husnara, in order to maintain Jamil's privacy.
(b)   You involve Husnara in her grandfather's care, so that you are able to communicate better with Jamil.
(c)   You leave without providing the care, as you hope you might be able to return with a trained interpreter at another time. You are not sure whether this will be possible.
(d)   Your action is different. State what you would do.

■■

In deciding what action you would have taken, these issues and questions may have been raised:

■   Is it acceptable to give care without asking permission, discussing or explaining this to a client?
■   Is it acceptable to involve a family member as an interpreter?
■   Is it ever appropriate to involve a child in translating for an adult?
■   Is it justifiable to leave care undone, whatever the reason?

Disclosing feelings

Carers have direct contact with clients and are often involved in personal and intimate activities such as assisting with washing or elimination. Clients sometimes make use of these situations as an opportunity to disclose their feelings, worries or fears.

Activity 5.8   ■■■■■■■■■■■■■■■■■■■■■■■■■■■■

Think of a situation where a client confided in you. Why do you think the client confided in you at that time? Make a list of all the factors you think made it easier for the client to communicate with you?
You may have included the following:

■   You knew the client well
■   You did not rush the client
■   The environment seemed more private.

What are the differences and similarities between your list and those of your colleagues? What positive elements are there from these collective experiences which could be applied as good practice in other situations?

If you are doing this activity on your own, it may be helpful to look at two or three of your own experiences and compare them.

■■

Working in an anti-discriminatory way

Every person, carer or client, is an individual with a set of values and views. As a carer it is important not to impose differing values or to act in a way which is judgemental.

Direct discrimination

There are two main types of discrimination: direct and indirect. Direct discrimination is where different groups or individuals are in a position where they are not being treated equally in an open and obvious way. An example of this is discrimination against people who have physical disabilities, if an environment has not been designed or adapted for ease of access. Some environments where care is provided still need to be adapted to accommodate special needs, such as creating toilets large enough to allow access for people using wheelchairs.

Indirect discrimination

Indirect discrimination is a less obvious and more subtle form of discrimination.

Examples of such discrimination could be carers from ethnic minority groups being allocated the most unpopular shifts on the ward, or receiving fewer opportunities to attend study days.

Discrimination Acts

Laws such as the Sex Discrimination Act (1975) and the Race Relations Act (1976) (you may want to find out more about these) which can be used to combat discrimination, exist. Social services and health authorities have policies such as equal opportunities and there are procedures such as how to process complaints. Despite such legislation, policies and procedures being in existence, discrimination in care environments and the workplace still exists. Discrimination continues to exist for many reasons, including ignorance, fear, tradition, and unchallenging attitudes.

Activity 5.9 ■

List as many areas as you can where you feel people can be discriminated against.

Your list may include age, culture, gender, race, religion, sexual orientation. Now think of a situation where you, a friend, a colleague or a client may have been directly or indirectly discriminated against. Briefly describe the situation. What were the feelings at the time? Apart from the person experiencing the discrimination, were there any other people involved? How was the situation handled? Was the situation resolved? What were the feelings after the experience? Looking back at the situation, are there any ways you think it could have been prevented or more easily resolved? Are there any useful strategies learned from the experience which could be applied in other cases of discrimination?

■■■■■■■■■■■■■■■■■■■■■■■■■■■■■■■■■■■■

Challenging discrimination

Challenging acts of discrimination, or at least presenting images of people in a positive way is a means of acting as an advocate. Carers act as role models to their peers. An example of this is using language which is not derogatory about individuals or groups, such as using words that are not ageist or sexist.

Activity 5.10 ■■■■■■■■■■■■■■■■■■■■■■■■■■■■

Below are some phrases which are ageist (used in a way which degrade, present older people in a negative way or are patronizing):

- ■ Dirty old man
- ■ Mutton dressed as lamb
- ■ Old wives' tale
- ■ Pair of old washerwomen
- ■ Old folk, old fogy
- ■ Sweet little old lady

Try to think of similar types of phrases and alternative phrasing that could be used instead. It may be a useful exercise to spend the next week observing what negative terminology is commonly used in conversation and in newspapers.

■■■■■■■■■■■■■■■■■■■■■■■■■■■■■■■■■■■

Deciding what action, if any, to take in everyday situations of conflict or discrimination is not easy. When caring for people, the work environment is not perfect and carers, clients and relatives do not always act or respond positively or in an anti-discriminatory way. Taking the time to look at the situation objectively, seeking insight from colleagues, and later reflecting on what happened are useful strategies to develop in handling difficult situations.

Activity 5.11 ■■■■■■■■■■■■■■■■■■■■■■■■■■■■■

In each of these imaginary situations try to:

- ■ Identify what type of discrimination may be taking place and against whom.
- ■ Describe how you would attempt to handle it.
- ■ Decide what action would be taken, and why.

(1) On the ward, Hugh, a 78 year old man, is visited by his partner

Charles. Hugh says to you they would like some privacy and wonders if the curtains can be drawn round the bed. Robert, in the same bay as Hugh, tells you he has seen Hugh and Charles holding hands and he objects. He says he wants to be moved out of the bay.

(2) Eileen has dementia, though at times she appears lucid. She asks to see the Roman Catholic priest urgently. It is Tuesday morning, and the priest is not due to visit the ward again until Saturday.

(3) Dorothy, a colleague says at handover that Mrs Dean has strongly expressed a wish to be cared for by 'white' nurses only, instead of 'black' ones.

■■■■■■■■■■■■■■■■■■■■■■■■■■■■■■■■■■■■■

Who best to advocate?

Deciding who would be the best person to act as advocate in a situation has the potential for contention. Sometimes clients are in circumstances that prevent them from being able to choose an advocate for themselves. There are no rules, and each situation needs to be examined individually. There are positive and negative aspects to different groups or individuals acting as advocates.

Carer's role

Carers are often in the position of knowing clients well from spending time with them. Carers are usually within a multi-disciplinary team and so may be able to use the skills they have in communication and negotiation on behalf of clients. Salvage (1987) states: 'Our first responsibility is to our clients, not to our colleagues, not to other health workers, and not to our employer'.

Clients are the focus of care. However, carers can find themselves in a vulnerable situation or in conflict with their employers as a result of high-lighting needs or 'whistleblowing' (reporting a situation where standards are felt not to be safe or high enough). Carers may be in situations where the everyday demands on them prevent them from being able to spend enough time to work effectively in an advocacy role. Often carers are in powerful positions compared with clients, and instead of working with clients to make decisions they may switch to making decisions for their clients, believing they know best. This patronizing approach, often done with the best of intentions, is called paternalism or maternalism, where the carer acts more like a parent with the client.

Family involvement?

Family and relatives are often close to clients and have the benefit of being able to draw on the history of a client's life and to be able to contribute to decision making, particularly where a person is suffering from dementia. However, since they are emotionally involved with the client, family and relatives may not be able to be clear or work objectively. Sometimes families have interests and priorities which are in conflict with the client, and so would be unable to work in a fully representative way as an advocate.

Independent advocates

Independent advocates, who are neither carers nor family, are another alternative. The advantages of such advocates are that they can work independently, outside structures like the NHS, and so are not vulnerable or held in check by employers. The disadvantages of such schemes are sometimes difficulties in gaining access to their services due to the demands placed on them. There is now a move to create advocate posts within a structure; this is very much tied in with looking at quality assurance and the demands of working towards the 'Patients' Charter' (Department of Health, 1992).

By the year 2025 the numbers of older people are expected to have increased dramatically. It is an ideal time to look at encouraging the development and expansion of self-advocacy, where groups and individuals work at becoming stronger and more effective in representing themselves.

Summary

Advocacy is an enormous subject, still needing much debate within care settings. Carers need to work openly in partnership with clients and regarding them as equal yet individual human beings. This is the most important concept to grasp at the point of care delivery.

References

Allen, R. (1989) (ed.) *The Oxford Dictionary of Current English*, Oxford University Press, Oxford.

Brown, M. (1985) Matter of commitment, *Nursing Times*, 1 May **81**(18), 26.

Carpenter, D. (1992) Advocacy. *Nursing Times*, 1 July **88** (27), 11.

Clark, J. (1986) Nursing Matters, patient advocacy. *The Times Health Supplement*, 19 February, 16.

Copp. L.A. (1986) Nursing Matters, patient advocacy. *The Times Health Supplement*, 19 February, 16.

Department of Health (1992) *Patients' Charter*. HMSO, London.

Goodwin, S. & Mangan, P. (1985) A guide to the stars, *Nursing Times*, 13 November **81**(46), 30.

Salvage, J. (1987) Whose side are you on? *Senior Nurse*, 6 February **6**(2), 20

UKCC (1989) *Exercising Accountabilty*, March, Section E (Advocacy on behalf of patients and clients), 12–13.

UKCC (1994) *Code of Professional Conduct*, June UKCC, London.

Wells, R. (1988) Ethics and information. *Senior Nurse*, June, **8**(6), 10.

Further reading

Age Concern (1986) *The Law and Vulnerable Elderly People*, Age Concern, London.

Aldbarran, J. (1995) Should nurses be politically aware? *British Journal of Nursing*, **4**(8), 461.

Cahill, J. (1994) Are you prepared to be their advocate? Issues in patient advocacy. *Professional Nurse*, March **9**(6), 371.

Centre Policy on Ageing (1995) *Citizen Advocacy with Older People, Code of Good Practice*. COP, London.

Chapman, A. *et al.* (1994) *Dementia Care; Handbook for Residential and Day Care*. Age Concern, London.

Cohen, P. (1995) Speaking up for others patients rights, *Nursing Times*, 29 March **91** (13), 54.

Dyer, S. (1994) Power to the people. *Elderly Care*, September/October **6** (5), 30.

Gates, B. (1995) Whose best interest? *Nursing Times*, 25 January **91** (4), 31.

Gwilliam, C. (1996) Dementia and social model of disability. *Journal Dementia Care*. Jan/Feb, **4** (1), 11.

Hart, J. & England, J. (1995) *Investing in the Heart of Change: The Case for Resourcing the Support of Self-help Activities*, NCVO, London.

Kenderick, K. (1994) An advocate for whom – doctor or patient? How far can a nurse be a patients advocate? *Professional Nurse*, March, 826.

Rich, S. (1995) Meeting the challenge. *Nursing Times*, 25 January **91** (4), 34.

Walsh, P. (1985) Speaking up for the patient. *Nursing Times*, 1 May **81** (18), 24.

Chapter 6
Elder Abuse
Jean Valsler

Overview

Older people can become the victims of abuse; therefore it is important that anyone who works with older clients is aware of the issues involved and clear about what to do if the problem arises.

This chapter provides an introduction to the subject of elder abuse. It first defines and gives details of the different types of elder abuse.

■ The identifying signs
■ Risk factors
■ Possible causes
■ Information is provided about the history and prevalence of the problem

The chapter is then devoted to looking at strategies for prevention and intervention. Guidance is given about the steps to be taken if elder abuse is suspected or witnessed. A brief summary is provided of the current relevant legislation and ways of offering ongoing support are also explored.

Throughout, there are activities to enable you to look at practice in relation to elder abuse in your own work and workplace.

Key words

Elder abuse, old age abuse, neglect, inadequate care, abuser, perpetrator, abused, victim, mental competence/incompetence, legal capacity/incapacity, confrontation, disclosure.

What is elder abuse?

There is no one all-embracing definition of elder abuse, but for the purposes of this chapter the following has been selected.

'Elder abuse is a single or repeated act or lack of appropriate action occurring within any relationship where there is an expectation of trust, which causes harm or distress to an older person.' (*Action on Elder Abuse Bulletin*, 1995)

The terms 'neglect' and 'inadequate care' are also frequently used in reference to the care of older people. These are less emotive expressions than 'abuse'. They can be useful in describing situations where the deprivation of assistance or care, which is necessary to the client's well-being has arisen not out of deliberate mistreatment by the carer, but because of unintentional failure to act on his or her part.

When the terms elder/older person or client are used in this chapter they refer to people over the age of 65.

Types of elder abuse

There are four kinds of abuse. physical, psychological, sexual and financial.

Where does elder abuse occur?

Domestic setting

- Person's own home
- Home of partner, relative or friend

Institutional Setting

- Residential homes
- Nursing homes } these can be in the local authority or in the private or voluntary sectors
- Day centres
- Day hospitals } NHS or private sector
- Hospitals

Who is abused?

Elder abuse crosses national, class, religious and cultural boundaries. Both men and women are abused. Older people who are physically and mentally fit are subject to abuse as well as those who are frail and dependent, although the latter group in certain situations may be more vulnerable, e.g. in cases of sexual abuse. The older person may not recognize that he or she is being abused but nonetheless abuse may still be taking place.

Who abuses?

The abuser is usually known to the older person and may be any of the following:

- Spouse
- Partner
- Son or daughter
- Other relative
- Friend
- Neighbour   These may be providing care but
- Acquaintance   this is not always the case
- Paid member of staff
- Volunteers
- Visitors
- Other patients or residents

In assessing situations of abuse it is important not to fall into the trap of stereotyping all older people as frail and helpless victims. They can also be capable of mistreating others and often abuse is not one-sided.

Abuse can be carried out by an individual or a number of people. In an institution it can be one member of the staff abusing an individual client in an otherwise well-managed establishment. Or it can be the entire work-force abusing all the clients because of attitudes and practices that fail to recognize the basic human rights of older people i.e. to have privacy, to make choices and to be considered as individuals.

How to recognize elder abuse

Anyone who works with older people needs to know how to recognize abuse. In order to do this it is necessary to develop an awareness of:

(1) *The signs* i.e. the indicators that elder abuse is occurring or has occurred.
(2) *The risk factors* i.e. the indicators that elder abuse could occur.
(3) *The causes* i.e. the reasons why elder abuse occurs.

What are the signs of abuse?

Some of the signs are indicative of more than one kind of abuse, and those relating specifically to physical, psychological and sexual abuse can also be indicators of underlying medical problems. It is therefore important to conduct a thorough medical examination, usually undertaken by a doctor, to rule out the presence of physical or mental illness before reaching the conclusion that the client has been abused.

The presence of any one or even several of the signs is not absolute proof of abuse. It is also important to note that abuse may be taking place even when there are no visible signs.

Physical abuse

This is the application of physical force and/or withholding of care which results in the older person experiencing pain or discomfort.
Examples include:

- Grabbing, shaking, pushing, pinching, hair pulling, burning
- Hitting with or without a weapon
- Excessive administration of drugs or alcohol
- Withholding food or drink
- Failure to supervise adequately
- Restraining the older person without his permission e.g. locking doors or blocking exits with furniture
- Failure to provide appropriate aids i.e. glasses, dentures, walking frames etc.

Signs of physical abuse

- Bruises in well-protected areas e.g. under clothes
- Bruises to the face, lips, mouths
- Burns e.g. from cigarettes
- Scalds e.g. from immersion in hot bath
- Unexplained lacerations or abrasions
- Hypothermia
- Dehydration
- Malnutrition
- Poor hygiene
- Excessive drowsiness
- Sudden weight loss
- History of inexplicable falls
- Fractures for which there is no explanation
- Wounds that are the shape of an implement that could have been used as a weapon e.g. buckle or rope
- Lack of necessary aids or equipment e.g. dentures, frames, glasses
- Signs of old untreated wounds

Psychological abuse

This is the deliberate imposition of mental or emotional stress on an older person by the use of threats, humiliation or some form of non-verbal behaviour.
Examples include:

- Patronizing behaviour towards older people either by an individual or an institutional regime
- Verbal abuse e.g. shouting, teasing, swearing, name calling, insulting, threatening
- Making the older person ashamed of some aspect of his behaviour over which he has no control
- Ignoring the older person or withholding affection from him
- Denial of privacy or imposition of physical or social isolation

Signs of psychological abuse

- Insomnia
- Change of appetite
- Weight loss
- Loss of self-esteeem
- Confusion

Physical and psychological abuse are often seen together. Both physical and psychological abuse are more likely to occur in the domestic setting where the older person and the carer are living together. The majority of abusers in these situations are the spouses or adult children. The victim is not always particularly frail and mutual abuse is quite common. In cases of physical abuse the abuser is more likely to dependent on the older person, or suffering from mental illness and in cases of psychological abuse there is usually a history of a poor relationship (Fig. 6.1).

Fig. 6.1 Abuse can be verbal.

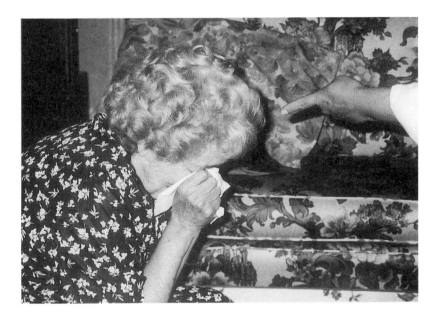

Sexual abuse

This arises when an older person is forced to endure sexual acts without his or her informed consent.

Examples include:

- Teasing
- Touching
- Kissing
- Caressing
- Molesting
- Rape

} without informed consent of the older person.

Signs of sexual abuse

- Bruising, pain, itching or bleeding from the anus, vagina or other genitalia
- Fingertip marks around the genitalia
- Difficulty in walking or sitting
- Onset of sudden confusion
- Reluctance on the part of the older person to be alone with the alleged abuser
- In a confused older person conversation can become overtly sexual and abuse may be spoken of as if it happened in the past when it is a current problem
- Bloody or stained underclothing
- Sexually transmitted diseases
- History of sexual abuse in the family or in the relationship prior to the onset of old age

Older people are not generally recognized as sexual beings, and as a result the fact that they can become victims of sexual abuse is often overlooked. Sexual relations between older people and others is quite normal providing both parties are consenting (see Chapter 3 Relationships). Older people can become the victims of sexual abuse whatever their sexual orientation. However, it appears from the little research that has been done so far that most victims are female and they are often physically or mentally frail. Most abusers are male and are usually living with the victim.

Financial abuse

This is the misuse of an older person's money or material possessions.
Examples include:

- Theft of money e.g. pension
- Borrowing money and not repaying
- Refusal to give the older person access to his or her money, property or information about them
- Cashing pension and not handing over the money
- Prevention of the delivery of necessary care on the grounds of cost

Signs of financial abuse

- Sudden inability to pay bills
- Sudden withdrawal of large amounts from accounts
- Disparity between income and living conditions
- Reluctance on the part of those administering the old person's money to spend it on services for which there is a fee
- Denying the older person choice as to how his money is spent
- Personal belongings going missing

Financial abuse is the most commonly reported type of abuse. The victims are more likely to live alone and to be socially isolated. The abuser is not always someone who is very close to the victim and he or she may have financial problems of their own.

Signs of abuse in the suspected abuser's behaviour

In assessing situations of suspected abuse it is important to be able to recognize signs that may be indicative of abuse in the behaviour of the alleged abuser. He or she may

- Have a poor relationship with the client
- Be aggressive to those who are trying to provide help
- Refuse others access to the older person
- Delay requesting medical help for the older person
- Be reluctant to permit older person to be interviewed alone
- Refuse to accept the rights of the older person
- Give a different account of events from that given by the victim and others

Any of the examples of abuse previously described can be found in either the domestic setting or in institutions. Here are some examples of abuses that are found in institutions where rules and regulations take precedence over individual choice and need.

Examples of elder abuse that can found in institutions

- Lack of respect for the individual's gender, sexuality or cultural and religious needs
- Rigid meal or bedtimes
- No choice of food/diet
- Lack of personal possessions e.g. shared clothing or toiletries
- Failure to provide choice of activities
- Lack of freedom to make phone calls/have visitors/to go out
- General lack of privacy e.g. no keys to own room, no lockable cupboards for personal possessions, staff opening the client's mail without his or her permission etc. (See Fig. 6.2)
- Lack of respect for confidentiality e.g. gossiping about the client's affairs either in or outside the institution
- Restraining the client without his permission e.g. locking doors, using cot sides etc.

Activity 6.1   ■■■■■■■■■■■■■■■■■■■■■■■■■■■■

Look back at the examples of abusive behaviours outlined. Make a note of anything either in your own practice with older people or within the structures/rules/policies of the organization for which you work that could be regarded as abusive to older people. Discuss your views with your manager and colleagues and try to find more appropriate ways in which to operate.

■ ■

Fig. 6.2 Denial of privacy and dignity is abusive.

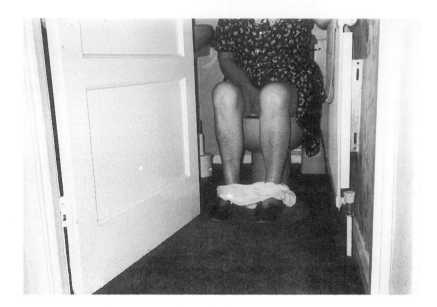

What are the risk factors in the domestic setting?

These are the indicators that there is a risk that elder abuse may occur at some point in the future.

There is a danger that abuse may occur in situations where a carer

■ Has undergone a change in life plans in order to take on the role of carer
■ Has multiple pressures
■ Feels he or she is being taken advantage of by other members of the family or the professionals involved
■ Feels he or she has difficulty getting others to recognize their needs
■ Is suffering from physical or mental illness
■ Often visits GP about his or her own health problems
■ Feels lonely and does not have adult relationships other than with the dependant
■ Does not get a break from caring
■ Regards the older person as being deliberately difficult where this is not the case
■ Frequently loses his or her temper
■ Admits to previously hurting the older person

Paid carers and volunteers in the domestic setting may be more likely to abuse if they are not trained and equipped to provide the level of care required and if they are not adequately supervised.

What are the risk factors in the institutional setting?

Abuse may occur in establishments where

- There is a poor atmosphere i.e. a sense of underlying tension between the staff or between the staff and clients.
- The management and staff spend most of their time away from the clients.
- The staff are more concerned with pursuing to their own interests e.g. rushing care tasks in order to attend to personal or staff matters.
- The staff are abused by the clients and this problem is not addressed.

The presence of any of the above risk factors in domestic or institutional settings does not mean that elder abuse will necessarily take place. These are warning signs that abuse may occur and as such must never be ignored but should prompt those involved to take steps to prevent the problem arising.

Activity 8.2 ■

 From your own work with older clients select two cases.

(1) The first should be one where there was a risk of abuse. Make a list of the risk factors that you observed.
(2) The second case should be one where the client was abused. Write a short paragraph giving details of the kind of abuse and the signs that indicated abuse was taking place.

Keep your notes for use later in the chapter where you will be looking at causes and methods of prevention and intervention.

■ ■

Why does elder abuse occur in the domestic setting?

Research into elder abuse is relatively recent and as yet the reasons it occurs are not fully known. It is likely that different types of abuse will have different causes.

Originally it was thought that elder abuse was most likely to arise in situations where a stressed carer was looking after a highly dependent older person. However many carers, even when extremely stressed, do not abuse their frail dependants. Where they do it is more likely to be a one-off or occasional expression of frustration than a pattern of sustained mistreatment.

Evidence shows that where there is ongoing abuse it is likely that the abuser is mentally ill or in some way dependent e.g.

- On drugs or alcohol
- On the client for emotional support
- On the client for accommodation and financial assistance

It is also clear that elder abuse is more common in circumstances where a poor relationship between the abuser and victim pre-dated the onset of old age. For example, a daughter who is caring for a father who abused her as a child may be at greater risk of mistreating him than one where abuse has not been a part of the earlier relationship.

Why does elder abuse occur in the institutional setting?

Elder abuse is more likely to occur in institutions where the approach adopted by staff has become depersonalized and dehumanized i.e. where the older client has become viewed more as an object than as a human being. This can happen when

- There is no stated philosophy or policy of care that recognises the older person's right to autonomy, privacy, and choice.
- There is no clear plan of care for each individual or system for monitoring and reviewing that care.
- Staff are untrained, low paid and have few career prospects.
- Staff have personal problems that are not acknowledged and addressed i.e. mental health problems, a history of being abusive.
- Management is remote and staff work in isolation.

Activity 6.3   ■

 What do you think the causes may have been for abuse arising in the cases you selected for activity 6.2? Make a note of your views.

■ ■

How much abuse is there?

It is difficult to be precise about the prevalence of elder abuse. Like other forms of abuse it is often hidden and therefore surveys may underestimate the size of the problem. There are a number of reasons why elder abuse is not always visible. For example, the abuse may go unreported if the older person

- Is mentally ill, e.g. with Alzheimer's disease and unable to recognize that he or she is being abused.

■   Is physically disabled/socially isolated and not able to summon help.
■   Has low esteem and does not recognize his or her right to be treated
     with respect.
■   The abuser does not acknowledge that he is abusing the older person.

Most research into the incidence of elder abuse has been conducted in
America and the findings are not necessarily an accurate reflection of the
problem elsewhere. There have been very few studies estimating the extent
of the problem in the UK. However, one study conducted in 1992 (Eastman,
1994) has shown that 'of the 593 people surveyed 32 (5%) reported having
been recently verbally abused by a close family member or relative 9 (2%)
reported physical abuse and the same number financial abuse.'

Sexual abuse has only been acknowledged as a problem for older people
relatively recently. It was not included in the above research but there is
sufficient evidence emerging from elsewhere to suggest it is an issue that
cannot be ignored.

Is elder abuse a new problem?

Elder abuse is not a new phenomenon; however it was only fully recognized as a social problem in the mid 1970s. The recognition of both child
and spouse abuse pre-date that of elder abuse.

The first type of elder abuse to be described was physical abuse.
Gradually the other types of elder abuse have been exposed, the most
recent being sexual abuse.

The USA has led the way not only in research but in developing specific
policies and procedures to deal with elder abuse. One of the first major
books on the subject in the UK was *Old Age Abuse* (Eastman, 1984)
published by Age Concern. Eastman's book served to stimulate interest in
the subject in the UK and this has slowly increased over the past decade
resulting in greater awareness and more research.

Research revealed that professionals were unclear about how to respond
when faced with cases of elder abuse. As a result, the Department of
Health recommended that all local authorities, in collaboration with other
interested parties, i.e. health authorities, the police and voluntary organizations for the old, compile local guidelines for action to be taken where
elder abuse is suspected in domestic settings. The recommendations did
not include abuse in institutions.

In 1993 Action on Elder Abuse was formed to promote changes in
policy and practice in elder abuse by raising awareness, education,
promoting research and providing information (see Useful Addresses).

Current developments for tackling elder abuse in the UK

There is still no specific legislation or national policy for tackling elder
abuse. The Law Commission has made a number of proposals for the

introduction of legislation to protect vulnerable elders and also suggested reforms of certain existing legislation such as that relating to the Court of Protection. These proposals are currently being considered.

The majority of local authorities have produced, or are producing, guidelines for staff. Unfortunately only a few of these have been drawn up with other agencies and most are not being monitored.

Action on Elder Abuse now runs an advisory service and publishes a bi-monthly bulletin updating its members on all matters relating to elder abuse in the UK and abroad.

Action to be taken in cases of elder abuse

Having established what elder abuse is and how it can be recognized, the next step is to look at what can be done about it.

In this section the following aspects of dealing with elder abuse will be examined.

(1) *Assessment* i.e. the investigative steps to be taken to establish whether there is a risk of abuse or evidence that it has occurred.
(2) *Prevention* i.e the steps to be taken to avert elder abuse
(3) *Intervention* i.e. the steps to be taken
    (a) to stop the abuse and to protect those involved
    (b) to offer ongoing support and to ensure that there is no recurrence of the problem

Aims and guiding principles for responding to situations of elder abuse

Before examining the different aspects of dealing with elder abuse it is important to be clear about the overall aims of work in this area. As stated previously, the victims of abuse have been deprived of basic rights and as a result they may be low in self-esteem and feel frightened. Abusers are also often vulnerable e.g. physically or mentally ill, dependent and/or burdened by feelings of guilt.

Therefore, the aims in working with those affected by abuse are

■ To protect the victim by preventing abuse or by stopping it at the earliest opportunity
■ To alleviate the effects of the abuse for those involved
■ To restore to the victim his basic human rights

The following are the guiding principles to be applied to ensure good practice in this area of work.

(1) *Take seriously all reports of abuse*. It is never appropriate to ignore the problem.
(2) *Treat all those involved with respect*. Elder abuse is a difficult area of

work and one that can arouse strong emotions in workers. It is not helpful to let these feelings show or to let them cloud judgement.

(3) *Remember that the victim is an adult* and as such is free to make decisions about how to live his or her life. This means that he or she has the right to take risks and may choose to continue to live in a situation that is abusive.

(4) *Seek the victim's consent before taking action on his or her behalf.* In certain instances an older person may be mentally ill to such a degree that he or she is not capable of making informed decisions. Then he or she may be deemed mentally incapacitated in the legal sense (see section on Legal framework below) and in such circumstances decisions can be made on his or her behalf. In such cases those responsible for making decisions should try to take into account what the older person would have wanted. It is rare that someone is totally unable to make any choices concerning their life and the client should be permitted to make those decisions of which he or she is capable and which do not place him or her at an unacceptable level of risk.

(5) *Intervene in the least disruptive and the least restrictive possible way.* While intervention should be designed to protect, it should also seek to empower the older person.

(6) *Respect confidentiality.* Many victims of abuse feel ashamed of what has happened to them. They and their abusers can find it very difficult to share information about the abuse with others. It is important that the victim's right to privacy in this painful and very personal area of the life be respected. Where the sharing of information with others is indicated, e.g. so that other professionals can conduct assessments or provide support, this should be discussed in full with the victim and his or her permission sought. Details should be given as to what information is to be divulged to whom and for what purpose. It should only be made available on a need to know basis and to those who are committed to maintaining confidentiality.

(7) *Do not adopt wholesale the procedures used to tackle other forms of abuse.* It is logical to ask if the procedures that have been developed for other kinds of abuse, e.g. child abuse and spouse abuse are applicable in elder abuse. There are some similarities between the various kinds of abuse and some lessons can be learned from experience in these areas. However there are also many differences which mean that specific approaches must be developed to deal with the aspects that are unique to the abuse of older people.

Assessment

The purpose of assessment

This is as follows:

(1) To establish whether there is a risk of elder abuse, or if there is evidence to suggest it has occurred.

(2) To gather information to determine what is the most appropriate form of intervention.

Who conducts the assessment?

Under the NHS and Community Care Act of 1990 local authorities have the responsibility to assess the needs of vulnerable older people. Therefore, the assessment of suspected cases of elder abuse will normally be co-ordinated by the social work department.

The assessment should be comprehensive and as such should involve the skills of a number of different professionals.

However, any worker who is made aware of a possible case of abuse has the responsibility to ensure that the situation is reported to those whose duty it is to conduct the assessment, even they are not personally involved in the process.

What knowledge/skills are necessary to conduct the assessment?

Those conducting the assessment need to know:

(1) The causes, risk factors and signs of elder abuse
(2) The local guidelines on elder abuse
(3) The relevant legislation
(4) Methods of interviewing
(5) The intervention and prevention strategies indicated for the different types of abuse
(6) The resources available and how to access them

Activity 6.4 ■

Do you know what is expected of you if you suspect or come across elder abuse in the course of your work? Obtain a copy of local guidelines for action in cases of elder abuse. Your manager should be able to advise you which guidelines are applicable to your area of work. If you do not have guidelines, use those provided here. Read the guidelines, together with the summary of relevant legislation then using your case examples from earlier in this chapter, work with your manager to clarify the following:

(1) Your role
(2) The responsibility of others ⎯⎯⎯⎯ in the assessment process

■ ■

Guidelines for action to be taken if elder abuse is suspected or witnessed

Taking the referral

Any worker who suspects, witnesses or is told of an abusive situation has a responsibility to collect as much of the information in (Table 6.1). as possible.

If the referral is being made by someone other than the victim, then it is important to establish whether permission has been given for the referral to be made. If permission has not been granted, the referrer should be encouraged to obtain it before taking the referral. If the referrer is not willing or able to do this, a referral should still be taken and discussed with the manager.

Table 6.1 Information required at point of referral

Re the abused
Name/address/tel.no/age/gender/ethnic background/language/religion/next of kin/other
Relevant contacts, i.e. relations, friends etc.
Details of physical and mental health/functional ability
Support network

Re the abuser
Name/address/tel.no/age/gender/ethnic background/language spoken/ relationship to the victim.

Re the abuse
Description of the abuse i.e. the type/details of evidence/how long it has been going on and how often it occurs and whether it is mutual or one-sided.

Re the referrer
name/address/relationship to the victim and the abuser if any/willingness to give evidence if required.

Consultation with line manager

The referral should be discussed with your line manager at the earliest opportunity even if all the above information is not immediately available. The purpose of the discussion is to determine what action should be taken and by whom.

For example:

- Refer to the social services department to co-ordinate the investigation in a case of abuse in a domestic setting. For example, where the alleged abuser is an informal carer, relative, friend or acquaintance.
- Refer to the relevant employers where the alleged abuser in the domestic setting is a paid member of staff or a volunteer.

■   In cases of abuse in an institution, refer to the manager of the establishment who has the responsibility to initiate an enquiry.

Assessment in the domestic setting.

Step 1   Planning the visit

The social worker or care manager appointed to co-ordinate the investigation should:

(1)   Gather further information, i.e. details of agencies involved and the nature of the contact together with any factors that have given those involved cause for concern in in the past.
(2)   Decide in conjunction with their line manager who should visit.

Options
It is also a good idea for two people to visit and interview the client and abuser separately, but care should be taken not to involve too many people as this can be overwhelming.

Ideally, one of the people should be someone who has a good relationship with the client and alleged abuser and to whom they may feel able to disclose abuse, e.g. a home help, district nurse or day centre worker.

If the alleged abuser or client is mentally ill it may be useful to have a doctor, CPN (community psychiatric nurse) or ASW (approved social worker) present. An interpreter should be present if this is required.

The police may be asked to attend, for example if there is a risk of harm to the workers involved.

(3)   Plan in advance of the visit with the co-worker (social worker or care assistant) and manager how to approach the interview.
(4)   Check access arrangements. For example, if the alleged abuser is the person who controls access to the older person it may be possible he or she will refuse admission to the people conducting the interview.
(5)   If appropriate, seek legal advice about access/intervention.
(6)   Notify the client of the planned visit.
(7)   It may be rare that there is a risk to the workers making the assessment but it is good practice and a wise precaution never to leave anything to chance. The details of address being visited and expected time of return should always be left with the manager.

Step 2   Assessment visit(s)

The victim should be visited and interviewed as soon as possible after the referral. The same priority should be afforded to elder abuse as to child abuse.

The client and the alleged abuser should be interviewed separately (see section on interviewing victims and abusers). The interviewers should look for the factors outlined in Table 6.2.

If at the end of the interview it is felt that there is a need for further investigations, e.g. by a doctor or the police, then the permission of the client should be sought.

Table 6.2 Information to be sought for assessment purposes.

Risk factors or evidence of abuse.
Details of circumstances that might have led or might lead to abuse.
The degree of danger to the client.
The client's and the alleged abuser's

(1)	Physical/mental health and functional ability	(5)	Support needs
(2)	Mental capacity	(6)	Support networks and apparent gaps in these
(3)	Living conditions	(7)	The levels of stress
(4)	Financial situation	(8)	Relationship with each other

It is often useful to ask about the daily routine as this can highlight problem areas.

Step 3   Discussion with line manager to decide on action

If there is immediate danger to the client then action to protect the client may need to be taken after the initial visit and a fuller assessment conducted once the client is safe. If there is no immediate danger then a comprehensive assessment can be conducted over a number of visits. A slower approach also enables the workers involved to build a good relationship with the client and carer.

Step 4   Case conference

A case conference should be called involving all the staff involved, the victim, and where appropriate, the abuser to decide:

(1) On the most appropriate means of prevention or intervention.
(2) Who will be responsible for providing help and to set dates for monitoring/reviewing the situation.

Assessment in the institutional setting

Step 1   The responsible manager should notify their own manager/ employers and plan a full enquiry.

Step 2   The client must be made safe during the investigation. Where the alleged abuser is a visitor or another client it is wise to try to separate them from the victim. If the alleged abuser is a member of staff a decision should be made as to whether they should be suspended pending the enquiry.

Step 3　The victim and the alleged abuser must be interviewed. Depending on the seriousness of the allegation it may be necessary to involve the police and if the client's needs require assessment the social services should be involved.

Step 4　The details of the enquiry should be recorded and the referrer, the victim and the alleged abuser informed of the outcome.

Step 5　The victim should also be given details of the appropriate authority to turn to if they are unhappy with the outcome.

Interviewing the victim of abuse and/or the alleged abuser

Both victims and abusers may be afraid and find it very difficult to admit to others that abuse has occurred. The task of all who work with older people is to try to make it easier for those involved to disclose what is happening. The staff who are responsible for assessing the situation should be skilled in conducting interviews and would normally undertake the task. However, the client and abuser may find it easier to talk to someone with whom they have regular contact and an established relationship. This could be a care assistant, day centre worker, district nurse, etc. Therefore it is important that all staff know how to encourage and facilitate discussion of abuse.

Activity 6.5　■ ■

Try to imagine that you are seeing a client you believe has been abused. How would you encourage him to disclose the matter?

■ ■

Points you should have considered are as follows:

Create physical space. Give the client control of the situation; if he or she is able, let him or her select the time and place, and whether to be accompanied by a friend or relative. The venue should normally be somewhere private where the client will feel safe and the interview will not be interrupted.

The interviewer should:

■ Remain calm and gentle in approach
■ Never hurry the meeting
■ Use language that the client can understand
■ Never push the client to disclose information until he or she is ready to do so
■ Never take sides or in dealing with abusers be punitive.

If disclosure takes place the interviewer should:

Thank the victim or the abuser for the information and acknowledge that it cannot have been easy to share this. Reassure the victim that the abuse is not his or her fault if this is their concern. Seek agreement about sharing the information with relevant parties.

If there is denial and this seems to be contradicted by the evidence the interviewer should:

Reiterate his concerns that he thinks abuse might be occurring. Encourage the client and/or the abuser to think over the situation and try to see him again to provide a further opportunity for the subject to be discussed. Try to find out what may be stopping the client/alleged abuser from disclosing and seek to allay these fears.

Prevention

The prevention of elder abuse should be a primary aim of anyone working with older people. The following are ways in which this might be achieved.

Those working with older clients should make it their responsibility to:

- Be knowledgeable about elder abuse, i.e undergo training/join Action on Elder Abuse to keep up-to-date with developments in this area.
- Educate those with whom they come into contact about the problem.
- Be vigilant, i.e. see clients and carers regularly and give them the time and space to express their needs.
- Seek medical advice and help for clients promptly.
- Work closely with other professionals/specialists to ensure that clients' and carers' needs are fully assessed and that they have access to all the help they require.

In the domestic setting

In the domestic setting those working with clients and carers should ensure that prospective carer/carers are made fully aware of the client's medical condition, prognosis and how it will affect his or her functional ability prior to moving into care. Details should also be given of any medication and possible side-effects.

Encourage both the client and the prospective carers to think about what will be involved. For example, the older person will be losing his or her independence and the carer's life may be more restricted.

Advise the carer to consider if he or she really wants to take on the responsibility of providing care. The carer may be doing it by default because an emergency has arisen or because of pressure from others, e.g. family and professionals. The carer should also be helped to think about his or her own needs, e.g. what will it mean for him in terms of his or her career, relationships, health, housing, finances, etc. If the carer suffers from a mental illness or drug or alcohol dependency he or she should be advised to get help. If there has been a history of a poor relationship between the client and the prospective carer, both should be encouraged to think carefully about whether it is advisable to enter into the new arrangement.

In existing situations of care in the domestic setting make sure that the carer whether family member, friend, professional or volunteer is given the opportunity and encouragement to say if he or she is running into difficulties. This can be achieved by giving the carer space and time to express his or her needs and by regular monitoring and reviewing of the situation. Also to provide the services and support needed.

Help carers avoid isolation by putting them in touch with self- help groups (see Useful Addresses). Advise the carer on the action to be taken if he or she feels they might abuse the older person. For example make the older person comfortable and as safe as possible. Get away to another room or outside. As soon as possible talk to someone about your problems such as a member of the family or a friend, or if these are not appropriate, to a GP or the social services.

In the institutional setting

In the institutional setting it is important that the staff are trained and equipped to provide the level of care required by the client. Any special needs that the client has must be taken into account, e.g. in the case of those from other cultural backgrounds attention will need to be paid to the language spoken, religious observances and dietary requirements.

In situations where the client has a disability, staff should be aware of the issues relating to that disability and both the client and staff provided with the appropriate support in terms of services, equipment and specialist advice.

Staff training and procedures

The management of the establishments should ensure that staff are given training to do the job and that they are supervised. Make sure that there is a clear system for monitoring and reviewing care as the needs of the client can change over time. Make sure that there is a clear and well-publicized complaints procedure. Ensure that staff are trained in how to handle complaints without becoming defensive. Make sure that the care of clients who exhibit difficult behaviour is shared. Ensure that staff have access to stress management training where appropriate.

Activity 6.6 ■

 Using your example of a case where there were risk factors devise a plan of prevention.

■ ■

Intervention

To date there are few proven methods of intervention in this area of work. It would appear that the intervention strategy will be determined by the degree of risk, the client's willingness to comply with the help available and also by the underlying causes of the abuse. For example, the response required where the cause of the abuse is carer stress and there is no immediate risk, is not the same as where the underlying problem is the carer's mental illness and there is a risk to the safety of the client.

The first objective of the intervention must be to protect the client. This is not always easy. On occasions a client who is mentally competent will persistently reject help and in such circumstances there may be little that can be done. If the client is mentally competent and agrees to intervention, or is mentally incapacitated and action can be taken on his behalf, then the first step may be to remove the client to a place of safety, i.e. a hospital if medical attention is required, or to a residential or nursing home. This has often tended to be the favoured option although it can prove to be disruptive to the already vulnerable client, and does not guarantee that the abuse will cease.

It may be better to consider removing the abuser. The law can be used if he or she is threatening or violent.

In situations where there is little immediate risk but where it is clear the abuser and victim need a break from each other then respite care or care in the home for the older person can be considered so that the carer can get away. The housing department can be approached if a more permanent separation is required and accommodation is the major issue.

If the client refuses help at this juncture it is important to try to maintain contact to give him an opportunity to seek help at a future date. It is also important to monitor that the situation does not get out of hand resulting in more harm to the client. Such monitoring should be regular and multi-disciplinary.

Once those involved are safe, it is important to implement a plan of action which will prevent a recurrence of the problem and seek to alleviate the distressing effects of the abuse.

In cases where carer stress is the main cause, the services provided to relieve the stress should aim to tackle the problem identified by the carer. It is of little use providing day care if the carer's primary concern is financial hardship. If isolation is the main concern, providing the carer with relief care and information of the various self-help groups may be useful.

In situations where the mental health of the carer or his or her dependency on drugs or alcohol are of concern then he or she should be encouraged and helped to seek appropriate medical advice.

Where elder abuse has arisen because of an established pattern of abusive behaviour in the relationship or family, counselling should be offered to both the abuser and to the abused.

Activity 6.7   ■

The above suggestions for intervention are not exhaustive. Using your example of a case where abuse occurred, make a plan for intervention and discuss with your manager and colleagues how this could be implemented.

■ ■

Legal framework

As yet there is no UK legislation that relates specifically to elder abuse. However, there are legal powers that can be used in a range of situations. Advice should be sought from the police or from lawyers where it is thought that legal action may be required.

Here there is only space to provide an explanation of mental incapacity and a brief summary of the laws that are relevant in elder abuse.

For those requiring greater detail, a particularly useful guide to the law as it affects older people in the UK is *The Law and Vulnerable Elderly People* (Greengross, 1986).

Mental incapacity

In assessing cases of alleged abuse one of the first points to consider is whether the victim and/or the abuser are mentally competent to make decisions because this to some extent determines what, if any, action can be taken on their behalf. Adults generally have the right to make decisions about their lives. The exception to this rule is where someone is deemed legally or mentally incapacitated or mentally incompetent.

This occurs when the law decides that someone is incapable of making a particular decision or engaging in a specific activity. For example, someone may be judged incapable of making a will or managing his or her finances on the grounds that he or she is suffering from a mental illness or mental impairment to such a degree that he or she is not able to understand what he or she doing.

Mental incapacity is usually determined by the use of a functional test and this is applied in most cases by a psychiatrist. If there is any doubt as to the client's mental competence a referral should be made to a psychiatrist for assessment via the client's GP.

Examples of relevant legislation

1   **Assessment and service provision**

■   *NHS and Community Care Act 1990 (Section 47)*

2   **To gain access where admission is refused**

■   *Police and Criminal Evidence Act 1984 (Sections 17/24/25)*

The police have the power to search premises without a warrant for the purpose of saving life or limb and to arrest any person who is suspected of having committed or is about to commit, an arrestable offence.

■   *Mental Health Act 1983 (Section 115)*
An ASW has power of entry and inspection of any premises, other than a hospital, in which a mentally disordered person is living if he or she has reasonable cause to believe that the patient is not under proper care.

■   *Mental Health Act 1983 (Section 135)*
This permits the ASW to apply for a warrant authorizing a policeman accompanied by an ASW and a registered practitioner to enter a person's home and if it is thought fit to remove that person to a place of safety on the grounds that he or she has been ill treated, neglected or is not being kept under proper control. or is unable to care for him/herself and is living alone.

3   Action can be taken in the following areas of abuse via the legislation listed

Physical abuse

■   *Offences Against Person Act 1861*
■   *Domestic Violence and Matrimonial Proceedings Act 1976*

Physical and/or psychological abuse

■   *Criminal Justice Act 1988 (Section 39)*
■   *Domestic Proceedings and Magistrates' Courts Act 1978*
■   *Race Relations Act 1976*

Sexual abuse

■   *Sexual Offences Act 1993*

Financial abuse

■   *Theft Act 1968*
■   *Power of attorney/enduring power of attorney* ⎱ can be used to
■   *Appointeeship*   ⎰ protect the
■   *Court of protection*   finances of clients

In exceptional situations where the victim is physically ill, frail or neglected, removal from home can be achieved via

■   *National Assistance Act 1948 (Section 47) and National Assistance Amendment Act 1951*
In cases where the victim or the alleged abuser are mentally ill, action can be taken in extreme circumstances to admit the mentally ill person to hospital via

■   *Mental Health Act 1983 (Sections 2, 3 and 4)*
Care can be provided in the community for certain mentally ill adults where it is in the interests of their welfare

■   *Mental Health Act 1983 (Section 7 Guardianship)*
The following legislation applies to abuse in the institutional setting

■   *Registered Homes Act 1984*
This gives the power to authorized staff of registration and inspection units to enter and inspect premises where vulnerable adults are living. All such homes must be registered either with the local authority or with the health authority.

Summary

This chapter has provided a basic introduction to the subject of elder abuse and by this stage you should:

■   Be able to recognize situations of potential and actual abuse
■   Be clear as to the action you should take if elder abuse is brought to your attention
■   Be in a position to assist in preventing abuse
■   Be able to assist in minimizing and monitoring abuse in the care setting
■   Know where to go for further information and support

It must be emphasized that this is only an introduction to the subject of elder abuse. There is much more information available and advances in this area of work are being made all the time. Those wishing to study the subject in greater depth are advised to undertake further reading and, if possible, attend training courses.

References

Action on Elder Abuse Bulletin (May/June 1995).
Eastman, M. (1994) *Old Age Abuse: A New Perspective.* Chapman & Hall, London. Co-published with Age Concern.
Greengross, S. (1986) *The Law and Vulnerable Elderly People.* Age Concern London.

Further reading

Abuse of Elderly People. Available from (with sae) The Distribution Service Dept, Age Concern England, 1268 London Road, London SW16 4EJ.
Eastman, M. (1984) *Old Age abuse.* Age Concern, London.

Bennet, G. & Kingston, P. (1993) *Elder Abuse: Concepts, Theories and Interventions.* Chapman and Hall, London.

Benson, B. (1995) *Elder Abuse,* Age Concern, Scotland.

Kingston, P. & Penhale, B. (1995) (eds) *Family Violence.* Macmillan, London.

Penhale, B. (1995) Recognising and dealing with abuse of the older person. *Nursing Times,* 18 October, **91** (42), 27.

Penhale, B. & Kingston, P. (1995) Elder abuse. *Health Care in the Community,* **3** (5), 311.

Wood, N. & Ford, M. (1995) Elder abuse. *Care Home Management,* 27 July, (59), 1.

Useful Addresses

Action on Elder Abuse
1268 London Road,
London SW16 4ER
Tel: 0181 679 2648.

Carers National Association
22–25 Glasshouse Yard,
London EC1A 4JS.
Tel: 0171 490 8818

Chapter 7
Supported Living
Helen Souris

Overview

'Give a man a fish, and you feed him for a day. Teach a man to fish, and you feed him for a lifetime'. (Chinese proverb)

This chapter considers the importance of encouraging your clients to remain as independent as possible within the limitations of their physical and mental health problems.

The move from a supportive to an independent environment is covered with an attempt to make you more aware of the possible difficulties that may confront the client. These include aspects such as mobility within their environment, management of domestic and personal resources, including finance, and the importance of maintaining contacts in potentially isolating situations.

This chapter also attempts to assist you to help the client overcome these problems through advice on intervention, assistive equipment and environmental adaptations.

Key words

Independence, mobility, assistive equipment, environmental adaptations, domestic resources, finance, social interaction.

Moving from a supportive to an independent environment

Planning the move

There may be many reasons accounting for an older person moving from a supportive to an independent environment. An improvement in an older person's physical and mental health may mean moving from a nursing or a residential home where most of their physical, mental and social care needs are being met by staff members, to living on their own. This may be their own home or sheltered accommodation which is warden controlled, but where they are essentially on their own. The most likely situation of a move from a supportive to an independent environment is however, discharge from hospital as a result of recovery from physical and/or mental health problems. Following a full assessment and treatment of their specific condition, it is hoped the person will progress to their maximum potential so that they can be discharged home.

Prior to discharge, it is important that the multi-disciplinary team (nurses, doctors, physiotherapists, occupational therapists and social workers), in conjunction with the client, draw up a plan for the client's future. An important aspect of planning for the future includes looking at accommodation. It may be that the client has made a full recovery and could return home, although a long period of hospitalization may have left the client with doubts as to whether they could manage on their own. There are, however, times when the client's illness has left them with residual problems.

Whatever the situation, it is important that the client is carefully assessed to determine a baseline for future action. The assessment should be a multi-disciplinary exercise in order that an accurate clinical judgement can be more readily achieved. It may be necessary for your client to have a Community Living Assessment.

Activity 7.1 ■

 Are you familiar with the Community Care Act 1990?

■ ■

The intention of the Act is to help people to lead, as far as possible, independent lives in their own homes. Clients should be offered the right amount of support and care, and a greater say in how they live their lives and to be able to discuss what services they need to help them to do so (Harding, 1994).

Through the administration of a Community Living Assessment, the client's needs are established, that is, their physical, psychological and social needs. Following presentation and approval at panels, decisions regarding a suitable environment are made, taking the client's wishes into careful consideration.

Activity 7.2 ■

 Familiarize yourself with the local policies and guidelines regarding Community Living Assessment in your work area, as the terms and procedures differ in each health authority.

■ ■

Whether the reason for hospitalization is as a result of physical or mental health difficulties, these problems will probably affect the person's ability to carry out activities of daily living. In order to determine the person's level of functioning, an occupational therapist may be requested to carry out an 'Activities of Daily Living' Assessment, or ADL. More specifically, assessment areas include:

(1) General level of functioning in self-care, domestic and practical activities

(2) Mental state cognitive functioning, orientation, memory and concentration
(3) Interpersonal functioning/social skills
(4) Level of awareness and insight
(5) Mobility and specific neurological problems.

The pre-discharge assessment should take place in the person's home environment to ascertain their ability to cope out of their present supported environment.

A development plan appropriate to the client's identified needs and stating the client's and others' role in implementing the plan is drawn up, agreed with the client, and recorded accurately. The necessary preparations for discharge are co-ordinated by the relevant members of the team. A keyworker is often allocated to the client whose role it is to do this; they work closely with the ward staff to ensure an effective and efficient discharge.

Activity 7.3 ■

Think about the aspects that need to be considered prior to discharge.

■ ■

You may have thought of some of the following:

■ Level of support in new environment
■ Present state of the environment
■ Basic essentials, that is, food, belongings and furniture, that need to be put in place
■ Informing people of discharge, that is, family, carers, warden, GP

Any change in a person's routine is bound to be unsettling and possibly frightening for the client, even though it is a decision that they have been actively involved in. It is important that team members and carers spend time with the client to express and discuss the fears and concerns which the client may have. Throughout this period, the carer's role is to give the client a lot of encouragement, reassurance and support; this may enable the client to overcome their anxiety and insecurities relating to the move.

Once they have moved to their new environment it is important that they are able to function independently and effectively within it. You need to ensure that your client is mobile and functional within their immediate environment and its surroundings. They also need to able to maintain their domestic and personal resources as well as manage money. They should be encouraged to take an active interest in local and community groups and events in order to prevent isolation and loneliness. All this may assist your client in coming to terms with the move and gaining in confidence to live independently.

Mobility within the environment

Maintaining mobility within the immediate environment

We all need to move in order to survive. Sometimes older people are prevented from moving as they suffer from an amalgam of different complaints. Their mobility difficulties may be as a result of physical frailty or disease, such as, arthritis, strokes or limited sight. They may also be because of factors which are not always immediately obvious, such as fear, distress and loneliness. For this reason, the approach adopted by the medical team and carers should be a 'holistic' one. Holism refers to the treating of the whole person including mental and social factors, rather than just the symptoms of the disease.

Whatever the reason for their mobility difficulties, this will affect their ability to move around in their own environment, and as a result their ability to maintain their independence (see Chapter 11 Mobility and Safer Client Handling).

Activity 7.4 ■■■■■■■■■■■■■■■■■■■■■■■■■■■■

What environmental factors should be taken into consideration when one's mobility is affected?

■■■■■■■■■■■■■■■■■■■■■■■■■■■■■■■■

Your list may include some of the following:

- Size of home
- Layout
- Whether the environment is easy to maintain
- Whether there are steps or stairs to negotiate
- What level or floor it is on
- Is it upstairs, is there a lift?

An assessment of the client's abilities and general layout by an occupational therapist can enable the client to continue living in their home by adapting the environment and providing assistive equipment and devices (Fig. 7.1). This may include measuring their homes for rails, raising armchairs to a suitable height and providing bathroom, kitchen and other equipment. There should be discussion and agreement with the client on environmental problems, and alterations should only be made after the client has proposed or agreed them.

Safety and security

Environmental adaptations and changes, as well as the provision of equipment is often not enough. Be aware of the general layout of the home. Is there enough space between items of furniture to ensure easy mobility of the person who walks with a stick, frame, trolley or wheelchair.

Fig. 7.1 Chairlift.

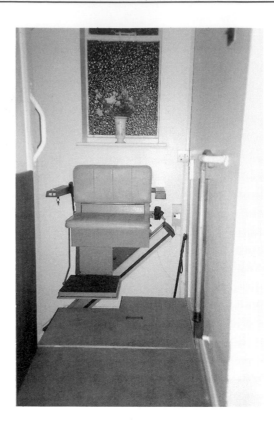

Non-slip, even floor surfaces are equally important. Mats and rugs that are loose, particularly frayed, can be dangerous. This problem can be overcome by securing them with double-sided sticky tape or drawing pins. Lighting should be adequate to avoid the client tripping and falling. It is important to encourage clients to ensure that decorations, furniture and fittings are safe and in a good state of repair and all appliances are operated safely.

Activity 7.5 ■

 The information discussed so far, relates to older people with physical or mobility problems. What difficulties do you think a person with dementia, that is, memory problems and confusion may encounter?

■ ■

When a person's memory fails, even a familiar environment may become confusing and frightening. A person may forget where their bedroom or bathroom is. This can obviously be very distressing for them. Labelling the different doors may assist them in orientation for place. Their safety throughout their home needs to be carefully considered. A common problem is a client's difficulty in remembering to turn the gas off. An alternative means of cooking may be a solution to this. Simplifying the environment may make it less confusing for the client with dementia.

Older people tend to be more vulnerable as they are often very frail, or may have visual or auditory problems. This will affect their ability to respond to intruders or unwelcome visitors. The client should, therefore, be encouraged and assisted to take appropriate measures to secure their living environment, that is, to lock doors, close windows and have methods of monitoring visitors. Your client should be aware of and informed of when and how to seek help on safety and security matters. As a carer it is important that you recognize potentially harmful situations or those considered most at risk. Raise your clients' awareness of risks and promote their ability to overcome them.

Preparation for a journey

It is not uncommon for an older person to become housebound. It may initially start off being as a result of poor mobility, and then later result in a disproportionate fear of leaving their home. Equally so, there are occasions when a person who is hospitalized and is ready for discharge, develops a fear of leaving the safe, secure environment of the ward.

It is inevitable that the person may have to go on a journey. If they are at home, this may include a medical appointment, day hospital, the shops or a social visit. As in the case of the person in hospital, a journey may include a home visit. It could mean an occupational therapy assessment to ascertain whether they are fit to go home, from a physical, emotional and social point of view.

Are you aware that your client has to consent to the journey? They may need to be prepared for the journey emotionally and psychologically, and possibly require a lot of reassurance and support.

Other preparations include the following.

Mode of transport and arrangements

- Are they travelling by *foot?* If so, are they aware of the distance to their destination? Do they have appropriate assistive equipment, footwear and clothes for the walk?
- *Manually powered vehicle*, such as bed, chair, trolley, stretcher, pushchair or wheelchair. Under these circumstances, the surfaces will have to be considered, are they flat? Are there ramps or lifts instead of stairs?
- *Motorized vehicle.* This could take a variety of forms depending on the circumstances.

Docherty & Harley (1987) review the different types of service available for transport depending on your client's destination and ability. These are:

- *Statutory* National Health Service, social services department and hospital transport.
- *Voluntary* Voluntary organizations using minibuses, local hospital car services.
- *Private* Private cars through relatives and friends; keep in mind that four-door cars are more convenient than two-door cars. The seats in two-door cars are difficult for rear passengers.
- *Independent* Use of public transport, although the associated problems may include high steps and awkwardly placed rails.

Clothing

Your client may require assistance in choosing appropriate clothes for the journey as well as help in dressing themselves.

Equipment

If the client uses mobility appliances, such as a walking stick, zimmer frame or wheelchair, these should be in good working order. Before making specific arrangements regarding the transport vehicle, ensure that the equipment can fit into the vehicle.

Accompanying clients on journeys and visits

You may be requested to accompany the client on such a visit. It is important that all transport details be negotiated with the client prior to the journey. This includes the client recognizing their need to be accompanied and consenting to it. When accompanying the client, reassurance should be given in such a manner to promote their sense of security, dignity and self-esteem.

Activity 7.6 ■

 What aspects would you as the escort need to consider when accompanying your client?

■ ■

Your list may include some of the following:

- Liaison with family members informing them of the impending visit.
- Support and reassurance – the client is often reluctant to leave their home or the hospital and may need a lot of encouragement to do so.
- Check whether medication or specific food need to be taken on the journey.
- Assistance with dressing ensuring that it is appropriate for the journey and visit.

Safety and security are of paramount importance. Ensure that all gas and electrical appliances are switched off, that the house is locked and your client has a set of keys with them.

The carer needs to be aware of any medical condition that may require urgent treatment; and methods of minimizing the different hazards which may occur during the journey.

Where the client uses mobility appliances, ensure that these are in good working order before use and removed for repair if not. These appliances may include wheelchairs, sticks, crutches and in some cases, prostheses and orthoses such as artificial limbs, braces and splints. Always use safe methods to assist clients into and out of vehicles.

Activity 7.7 ■

 Are you familiar with the legislation or organizational policies relating to transporting and accompanying clients?

■ ■

Legislation regarding transporting and escorting clients relates to clients that are hospitalized. If the client is an informal or voluntary psychiatric patient, and they wish to go on a journey and be accompanied, then all that is required is the consent of the client. If the client's mental health problems renders them at risk, the nurse in charge may suggest that they be accompanied by a member of staff, sometimes a carer.

The client may have been sectioned under the Mental Health Act 1983, that is, compulsory admission to hospital as a result of mental illness. Under these circumstances the client cannot voluntarily leave the hospital. Should the client need to go on a journey, they may be granted leave of absence from hospital under section 17 of the Mental Health Act of 1983. The responsible medical officer (RMO) is authorized to grant leave of absence for a specific period. The decision, which cannot be delegated to another professional, rests with the patient's RMO after necessary consultation. It is necessary in the interest of the patient or for the protection of others, that the RMO may direct the patient to be kept in the custody of another person. This may be any officer of the hospital staff or any other person authorized in writing by the managers of the hospital. It is under these circumstances that you may be requested to accompany the client, and you should therefore be familiar with this legislation.

Assisting occupational therapists in the provision of support and equipment to clients and carers in the community

Role of the occupational therapist

The role of the occupational therapist is to promote the client's independence within their limitations. The philosophy inherent in occupational

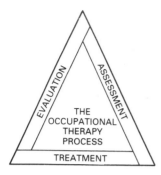

Fig. 7.2 The occupational therapy process.

therapy is to view the client holistically, taking into consideration their psychological, physical and social needs (Fig. 7.2).

The need for assessment may arise from:

- A referral from another member of the care team
- The client moving into the community after being in hospital or residential accommodation
- The client or carer making direct contact with the service

It is essential that carers have some basic knowledge of support and equipment that can be provided in the client's environment. To begin with, the client's needs should be established through communication and observation. This information should then be passed onto the appropriate professional, usually an occupational therapist who will do their own detailed, professional assessment.

A full occupational therapy assessment should be administered to determine what the client's abilities and limitations are and how these are impeding their functioning. The assessment areas that an occupational therapist covers have already been covered in the previous section. Blair & Glen (1987) identify the principles around which occupational therapy treatment revolve, these are:

(1) Attention to the total life-style and support systems
(2) Reinforcing residual assets and skills
(3) Adapting situations and the environment to minimize dysfunction
(4) Acknowledging psychological needs of the client and carer

If the client is in hospital or in a setting where there is an occupational therapist available, a therapeutic activity programme may be designed to treat the areas in which the client is experiencing difficulties. At home, the occupational therapist may give advice on modifications to the environment and assistive devices and equipment for activities of daily living. These will achieve the highest level of independent functioning within the limitation of the illness, and will in turn serve to relieve the carer.

Activity 7.8 ■

 Familiarize yourself with some of the environmental modifications and adaptive equipment that may enable your client to become more independent, and safer within their own home.

■ ■

In the *kitchen*:

- Broad-handled cutlery for easier grip (Fig. 7.3)
- Non-slip/dycem mats

- Kettle tipper
- Jar openers

Fig. 7.3 Adapted eating utensils.

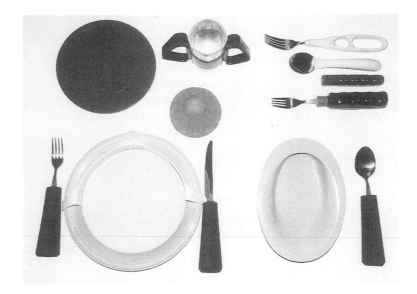

In the *bathroom*: (Fig. 7.4)

- Wall-mounted grab rails
- Raised toilet seat
- Bath seats
- Bath boards
- Bath mats
- Tap turners
- Long washing aids

Fig. 7.4 Adapted bathroom.

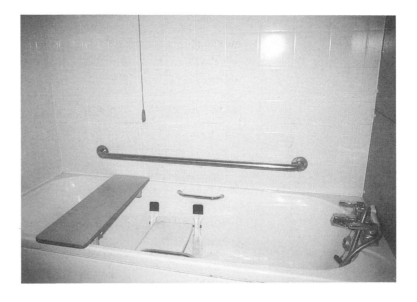

Dressing

- long-handled brushes and
  combs (Fig. 7.5)
- button hook (Fig. 7.6)

- tights aid
- shoe horn
- zip puller

Fig. 7.5 Aids to
independent hair care.

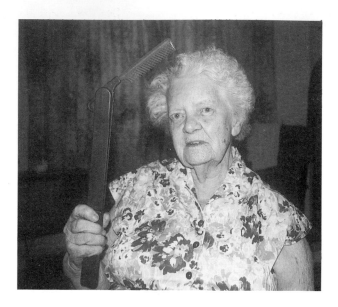

Fig. 7.6 Aids to
independent dressing.

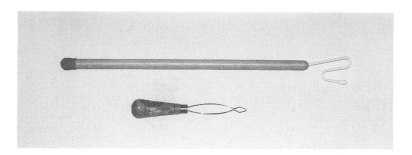

Miscellaneous:

- Easi-reach/reacher (Fig. 7.7)
- Chair/bed raisers

- Stair rails
- Key turner

Prior to any changes being made to the environment, the options and
information on support and equipment are explained in a manner and at a
level and pace, appropriate to the client and their carer. Following this, the
appropriate form of consent is obtained from those concerned.

Once the environmental modifications have been made (and how to use
them demonstrated), and the equipment given to the client, any difficulties

should be discussed with the client and possible solutions suggested. Should any problems arise at a later stage, this should be passed onto the appropriate professional without delay.

Managing domestic and personal resources

Personal clothing

Clothes fulfil many functions. They may keep us warm or cool and may assist in maintaining individuality. This is particularly pertinent to older people that have chosen continuing care and do not have their own homes to reflect their own identity. Clothes should be attractive enough to maintain their self-esteem and to encourage them to go out, since many clients are in a potentially isolating situation living on their own. Clients should be encouraged to select, wear and care for their own personal clothing to the greatest extent within their limitations. Should they encounter difficulties in dressing, it is important that everything be done to minimize their problems.

Activity 7.9 ■

Think about what problem areas may arise in the elderly in relation to clothing.

■ ■

Your list may include limited range of movement as a result of arthritis or cerebro-vascular disease. Also involuntary movements can cause problems for the client. Tremor is one of the commonest involuntary movements in older people. Other problem areas when dressing that arise in the elderly include:

- Breathlessness
- Incontinence
- Sensory loss
- Visual handicap
- Confusion
- General mobility

Maclean (1987) identifies how these problems can be overcome.

(1) Use different dressing strategies such as dressing the affected side first as in cerebro-vascular accident. Lean the elbows on a table to decrease flexion and abduction required at the shoulder joint so that the client can put garments over their head when the upper limb is still (Fig. 7.8).
(2) Make alterations to clothes. Remove buttons, zips and hooks and replace them with velcro. Increase the size of an opening or fastening, for example, use larger buttons and increase existing buttonholes.

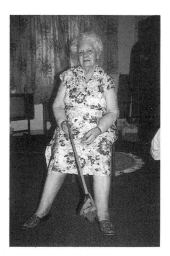

Fig. 7.7 Easi-reach/ reacher.

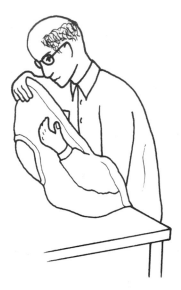

Fig. 7.8 Client with limited movement dressing.

(3)   Make use of dressing aids such as stocking aids, long-handled shoe horns, dressing sticks and button hooks (Fig. 7.9).

(4)   Choose or buy suitable garments, such as trousers and skirts with elastic waistbands. Choose clothes that are appropriate for age and life-style and comfortable in terms of fabric, style, size, appearance and acceptability to the wearer. The elasticity of the fabric should be non-constricting and the texture of the fabric must provide maximum comfort and be durable.

Care of clothing

Laundry of clothing can be particularly difficult for older people especially those with problems such as incontinence and food spillage. A washing machine is the ideal and easiest way, but not all older people can afford one. When purchasing garments the type of fabric and ease of cleaning should be considered. In addition to this, prewash soaking may decrease the time spent washing clothes and short spins or drip drying may decrease time spent ironing. Emphasize the importance of personal hygiene and keeping clothes clean. If the client is unable to do so themselves, ensure that soiled or infected linen and clothing is placed in the appropriate place and that your own personal protection and hygiene is maintained (refer to Chapters 9 and 10).

Activity 7.10 ■

    What safety issues need to be considered when choosing garments?

■ ■

- ■ Garments should be flame resistant
- ■ Garments should have no hard seams that may cause abrasions
- ■ Garments should not be slippery
- ■ Garments should not have loose ties and belts that may get caught when walking or transferring to a vehicle, etc.

Choice and preparation of food

Food is essential to all of us and is important for our physical and mental well-being. It is essential to ensure a person gets adequate nutrition. This is of particular relevance in the older person, who may over the years have developed physical aliments or illness and is dependent on a healthy diet to maintain their health (see to Chapter 8, Nutrition for the Older Person).

Encourage the client to choose food which is consistent with their preferences, personal beliefs and clinical needs. All their needs should be recognized and respected. Assist the client with any preparations that may be necessary. This may include making decisions regarding the menu, working within their financial budget, planning the journey to obtain the items and then finally the preparation of the meal itself. Preparing, cooking and storing the food should be done in ways which promote food appeal, maintain hygiene and minimize the risk of accidents.

Hygiene requirements can be met by complying with the Food Safety Act 1990. This Act relates to food hygiene and the preparation and provision of food.

Activity 7.11 ■■■■■■■■■■■■■■■■■■■■■■■■■■■

Familiarize yourself with the Food Safety Act 1990.

■■■■■■■■■■■■■■■■■■■■■■■■■■■■■■■■■■

The following principles can be used as a guide to safe practice:

- Ensure hands are washed prior to handling and serving meals.
- Wear a clean, disposable plastic apron so as not to contaminate food being handled.
- Any cuts or abrasions on hands should be adequately covered.
- Work surfaces, cooking utensils and equipment must be kept clean.
- Ensure food is adequately stored to minimize the risk of contamination, by storing it in the refrigerator below 5°C, and keep it no longer than the instructions on the label; or covered and sealed if appropriate.
- Waste food should be disposed of in a dustbin with a lid.
- Reheating food should be discouraged.

Obtaining household and personal goods

The client should be encouraged to identify shopping and supply requirements and to establish how these will be obtained. The client needs to be assisted with the preparation of the shopping list. They should work out their expenditure and budget allowance as independently as possible. Preparations relating to the journey should be carefully planned and the transport arrangements taken care of.

This framework can be applied to access any available services and information. The services may be financial, legal, religious, recreational, leisure, educational, training, health, social welfare, or everyday living tasks, such as shopping as mentioned above or launderettes. The client should be encouraged to make use of these services and facilities and the relevant information regarding these services should be obtained and preparations carefully made before going out.

Activity 7.12 ■■■■■■■■■■■■■■■■■■■■■■■■■■■

Imagine you are caring for an older person with mental health problems, such as dementia, depression, anxiety or bereavement. Imagine caring for someone with poor mobility as a result of severe arthritis. How might this affect their ability to carry out the domestic and personal activities

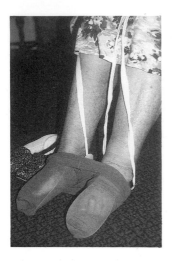

Fig. 7.9 Stocking aid.

such as food preparation, shopping and finance, etc. and how can these difficulties be overcome?

■■■■■■■■■■■■■■■■■■■■■■■■■■■■■■■■

You may have considered some of the following aspects:

Dementia

As a result of their poor memory, your client may be confused and disorientated in their own home. Making adaptations to the environment, for example, simplifying the layout and putting signs on the doors indicating which rooms the doors lead to, may alleviate some of the distress caused by disorientation.

A shopping expedition, or any other visit, will require careful planning and preparation. The client will need a lot of assistance in drawing up a shopping list, everything will have to be written down. It may be that the client's financial affairs are already being taken care of by their health care worker or yourself, and they will, therefore, require your assistance to work out what budget is available to them.

They will need to be accompanied on their expedition for safety reasons, that is, to ensure they get the right transport to their planned destination and that other people do not take advantage of their finances.

Depending on the severity of their memory, they will probably need a lot of assistance in meal preparation. As a result of their confusion and poor sequencing abilities, instructions will have to be written down in a logical order and each step verbalized, so that they are receiving visual and auditory cues. Do not have the expectation that your client will be able to learn new skills. If they are unable to use the cooker, the likelihood of them learning is remote. Ensure their safety by checking that they have turned their appliances off, particularly gas appliances. If your client is thought to be a risk to themselves and others, environmental adaptations, for example, switching the gas off may have to be considered. If your client rejects this or continues to be a risk in other ways, for example, wandering or neglecting personal hygiene, forgetting to eat or drink, etc. an intensive care package or alternative accommodation may have to be considered.

Depression, anxiety or bereavement

Many older people experience the loss of a spouse, partner or companion. In this situation they need time to re-familiarize themselves with basic coping abilities. When dealing with this client group, be aware of how these difficulties may have manifested in low self-esteem, dependency and lack of identity. An activity programme to help overcome these difficulties can involve talks from dieticians about special diets, low-priced meals or the nutritional value of different foods. Domestic activities should be graded beginning with simple snacks, such as making tea and toast to eventually organizing small lunch groups. Be aware of hazards in the home, using

COSHH leaflets (Control of Substances Hazardous to Health) and discuss possible potential safety hazards in the environment.

Initially, these clients may need to be accompanied on shopping expeditions to help them overcome their anxiety regarding this task. A discussion of money management, that is basic shopping, prices, pension, benefits and paying bills should be included (Blair & Reynolds, 1987).

Poor mobility

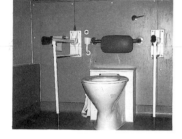

One of the commonest of all chronic diseases in older people is arthritis. this is a degenerative joint disease in which there is a progressive loss of function, resulting in poor mobility. In order for this person to remain independent and to continue managing domestic and personal tasks, the following has to be considered:

- Adaptations to the environment and provision of equipment that will decrease pain and ensure the protection of affected joints.
- Transport for shopping will have to be carefully planned and well organised.
- If the person has the assistance of a wheelchair, environmental factors such as ramps, wide doorways, lifts and disabled toilet facilities will have to be researched beforehand (Fig. 7.10).

Fig. 7.10 Aids to independent toileting.

Administration of financial affairs

As a carer, you may have to assist clients in the administration of their financial affairs. Clients should be encouraged to control their own budget and exercise freedom of choice. The client's payment obligations are ascertained and then the client is encouraged to pay these by their preferred method. This may be by cheque, standing orders, giro, cash or credit cards. Clients are encouraged to request receipts and to query any discrepancies. Should the client be unable to manage their own affairs, in the case of mental health problem or mobility difficulties, then they may allocate this task to the carer. In this situation where the carer makes payments on the client's behalf, they must ensure that the details are recorded accurately, legibly and completely following payment and in accordance with any required procedure. Ensure that the client's finances remain confidential, and are only disclosed to those agreed by the client.

Do you know?

There are existing administration policies/procedures which affect handling other people's finances.

The following will be covered briefly, but you should be aware of them as they may be relevant to you as the carer.

Agency

A person who receives a benefit or a pension may nominate someone called an 'agent' to collect the money for them, but not to spend it. The person entitled to the benefit completes the declaration on the reverse of the pension order to enable someone to collect the money for them.

Enduring Power of Attorney (EPA)

This is a legal document by which someone appoints one or more persons to act for them, should they in the future become incapable of managing for themselves. It must be executed and signed by the person while they are capable of understanding the nature and effect of creating an enduring power. The EPA should then be signed by an attorney as soon as possible while the person is still well. As soon as the attorney has reason to believe that the person is becoming mentally impaired, the attorney must apply to the Public Trust Office (formerly known as the Court of Protection) to have the EPA registered.

Public Trust Office

If an Enduring Power of Attorney has not been made, then the only way to manage the financial affairs of a person who is unable to do so for themselves would be to apply to the Public Trust Office. This is an office of the Supreme Court which exists to protect and manage the financial affairs and property of people who, because of mental disorders cannot manage for themselves.

The court can authorize the administration of the client's affairs by appointing someone to manage the patients affairs. The Public Trust Office would only become involved if something needed to be done either to protect the patients assets or to enable them to be used for the client's benefit.

Benefits and allowances

The client should be encouraged and supported to find out from an appropriate person the benefits and allowances that they are entitled to and information regarding the documents that need to be filled in to enable them to claim these benefits. The client should then be supported to complete the relevant details on the claim documents, so that they are complete, accurate and legible for submission.

Activity 7.13 ■

 Are you aware of some of the benefits and allowances older people are entitled to? Familiarize yourself with them so that you can ensure your clients receive them.

■ ■

Retirement pension

To qualify for the state retirement pension the client must have reached pension age (60 for women, 65 for men) and fulfil the National Insurance (NI) contribution conditions. The client is entitled to receive an extra 25p when they reach the age of 80, and may also receive extra pension if they defer drawing from their pension.

Income support

This is the social security benefit which is intended to help people who do not have enough money to live on and whose savings are below £8000. If your client qualifies for income support, they may also get other benefits such as the automatic right to free dental treatment, eyesight tests etc.

Attendance allowance

This is for people with severe disabilities, either for physical or mental health reasons and who have required regular attendance for at least six months. If the client needs the attention of someone on a regular basis, whether the help is from a neighbour, relative or private carer, then it is worth applying. Examples of attendance could be: assistance with washing, dressing, bathing, drinking or eating, assistance in getting up or going to bed, going to the toilet or assistance to move in bed. The difficulties may be as a result of mobility or physical difficulties, or as a result of cognitive impairment as in a dementing illness.

Before the allowance can be made, an independent doctor must come to assess the client's needs. The doctor is not there to check that the client is actually receiving care, but to ensure that they need the attendance of another person. Assessments by doctors vary and consequently it is always worth encouraging your client to appeal if they are refused the allowance. The allowance is paid to the person who needs the attendance to spend as they see fit. Perhaps it is best to see it in terms of an allowance to defray some of the expenses the client incurs because they need the attention of another person.

Disability living allowance

This allowance is for people who are unable, or virtually unable to walk. It also includes people who suffer with visual and hearing impairment. An application for this has to be made before the client reaches their 66th birthday and needs to show that they had these limitations before they reached the age of 65 years. This allowance will continue without an age limit as long as one satisfies the conditions. It requires an independent doctor to assess eligibility. It is paid to the client/claimant and it is intended to help with extra transport costs, but can be used as the claimant sees fit.

Invalid care allowance

This is an allowance for carers of working age who look after a disabled or frail person at least 35 hours per week. They are unable to work full time because of the care they are giving the client. The disabled person must be receiving the attendance allowance. This allowance is taxable and is affected by other income the carer receives. The carer must be over 16 and under 65 years when they claim in order to qualify.

It is also worth enquiring about *Housing* benefits and *Council Tax* benefit, as there are circumstances that your client may get a reduction.

Free NHS services include hearing aids, chiropody, prescriptions to women aged 60 or over, or men aged 65 or over. Those on income support are also entitled to assistance with dental care and optometry costs.

Once the benefit has been approved, the carer should encourage and support the client to claim and collect the benefits and allowances within the limited timescales. Any discrepancies should be reported. Money received should be kept in a safe and secure place.

A list of useful names of organizations offering help on legal and financial issues is provided at the end of the chapter.

Maintaining contacts in potentially isolating situations

Many older people live alone and are isolated. The factors which cause clients to become potentially isolated may be limited mobility, as well as mental health difficulties such as depression, anxiety, phobias and dementia. As a result of this, social contacts are limited and this in turn may have a profound effect on the individual and their relationships.

Encourage your client to express their need for and interest in maintaining social contacts. Establishing recreational and leisure activities will enable the person to gain contacts. If your client has just been discharged from hospital, you will need to consider their leisure interests and activity prior to admission as well as their present ability to participate and possible restraints.

Nystrom as cited by Blair (1990), divided activity patterns and leisure concepts among older people into:

■ *Passive* where the participant brings the world to them, for example, reading, watching television, caring for plants, listening to the radio;
■ *Active* going to the world by visiting relatives, attending clubs, going to church or entertaining friends.

He saw the need for options and choices of activity so that, if one activity was restricted due to physical or mental ill health, an alternative could be sought.

Many older people that live alone and are isolated may use their dependence on others as a means of gaining social contacts. They need encouragement and reassurance that becoming more independent may give them the opportunity to develop more contacts by becoming more mobile, and in turn, leaving their home and engaging in activities.

Explore the opportunities, together with your client, looking at the various options. Investigate clubs, church-based activities, libraries, community centre groups with the client to stimulate their interest.

Activity 7.14 ■■■■■■■■■■■■■■■■■■■■■■■■■■■

When looking at the options with your client, what practical aspects need to be considered?

■■■■■■■■■■■■■■■■■■■■■■■■■■■■■■■■■■

You may have thought of some of the following:

- Your client's interests
- What is available in the area
- Where it is possible to access information from differing services
- Whether transport is available, or whether it has to be organized
- Whether the outing/centre will meet the needs of your client

It is often helpful to accompany your client on their outing the first time they go, for example, to a day centre, as they may not have the confidence to go on their own.

Intellectual stimulation is also considered of great importance in the older person. Lewis as cited by Blair (1990), firmly believes in encouraging the older person to continue learning. Intellectual incompetency is not necessarily a natural phenomenon of later years. Where an older person has functional mental health problems and their mental state is improving, investigating community education centre, and the possibility of attending evening classes, can be incorporated as part of the rehabilitation schedule.

Where there is a danger that your client will lose a sense of purpose or interest in an activity, the information is passed to an appropriate person without delay. It may be that your client is depressed and has lost the inclination or motivation to become involved in activity. An assessment and treatment of their mental state by the mental health team may improve their mood and in turn their participation in social activities. The ability to adjust satisfactorily to ageing seems to be largely dependent on continued involvement in activity which gives a sense of purpose and enhances one's self-esteem.

Carer support

The term carer is used to describe a person who looks after an elderly, disabled or ill relative or friend who cannot manage on their own at home.

Carers can be children, partners, friends or neighbours (*see* Chapter 13 Caring for Carers).

The times at which support may be initiated varies. It may be at the stage of:

- Diagnosis of an illness
- Change in the client's condition
- On referral from the care team

Most of the literature to date has shown that caring for the elderly with mental health problems is stressful and leads to psychological distress in carers.

It is essential that the importance of the carer and their needs are acknowledged. Often one becomes preoccupied with establishing a relationship with the client, in turn neglecting the carer. The carer may need to talk about their frustrations at being tied to the elderly person and their fears and anxiety about their ability or strength to carry on. Recognizing the needs of the carer and supporting them may be important in the overall success of the situation. A carer may need to work very closely with a friend or relative. Their roles will probably largely overlap, so communication regarding expectations of the carer should be established from the start in order to avoid conflict.

Activity 7.15 ■

 What difficulties or concerns do you think a carer may encounter while looking after an elderly person with dementia?

■ ■

Your list may include some of the following:

- Lack of understanding of illness, management and prognosis;
- Anxiety regarding the client's safety, for example, wandering, leaving gas on, falls;
- Anxiety regarding own health, and who will care for the person if they get ill;
- Adjustment from previous life-style and relationship with the person they are now caring for which may result in social isolation and accompanying loneliness;
- Behavioural difficulties, such as, aggression, sleep disturbance, inappropriate sexual behaviour;
- Living bereavement – carer goes through the grief reaction as the person they knew and loved is no longer the same;
- Financial difficulties as they are often no longer able to work;
- Frustration of continually being asked repetitive questions;
- Fear of being left to cope without adequate support or help;
- Fear of watching their loved one decline in health;

- Fear of death of their loved one;
- Continually feeling tired and exhausted as a result of caring.

Carer intervention

Counselling and education

This will be from a professional person, to enable the carer to learn more about the illness, management and prognosis. The sessions will give the carer the opportunity to express feelings of anger, guilt, sorrow, frustration and aggression. This in turn can release pent-up emotions and help carers to cope with different stages of the illness and their reaction to it.

Carers' support groups

These groups give carers the opportunity to share similar experiences, which often alleviate a feeling of isolation. Some carers find that they can benefit from others' ability to cope with stress and learn from them. There is often an exchange of problems, a sharing of possible solutions and ways of coping. Occasionally, carers' support groups are held within a hospital or day hospital environment – this may give carers the opportunity to speak to different members of staff on specific problems.

Respite care

Respite admissions give relief to carers whose mental and physical state deteriorates as a result of continuous stress, lack of sleep and many everyday problems. Clients that have long term physical or mental health illness are most in need of this service. Clients may go into hospital, residential or nursing home settings usually for a period of two weeks, but this varies depending on the setting and the need of the client. Respite care enables the carer to look after the client for much longer.

Crossroads

This is a respite scheme which enables the carer some free time to rest or pursue their own interests or leisure activities, while the client is being well cared for by other carers. The service is usually available for a few hours each week, but can be extended into the evenings or the weekends if there is a big need.

As a health care worker, be sensitive and acknowledge the needs of others. It is essential to be aware of the services available to carers. Encourage them to make use of these services, as this may alleviate some of their stress, and in turn, ensure more effective and efficient care of the client.

Summary

This chapter has dealt with the importance of maintaining independence in all aspects of daily living, regardless of the existing living environment.

References have been made to various legislation and organizational policies that may be relevant in the effective care of the client.

It is hoped that the information and activities discussed enable the carer to gain insight into the difficulties experienced by the older person. It explores the ways in which a carer can assist these individuals in overcoming these obstacles in order to elicit their full potential, so that they may live a happy and meaningful life within the context of their illness.

References

Blair, S.E.E. & Glen, A.H. (1987) Psychiatry in old age: occupational therapy and organic conditions, in *Occupational Therapy with the Elderly*. Helm, M. (Ed.) Churchill Livingstone, Edinburgh.

Blair, S.E.E. & Reynolds, R. (1987) Psychiatry in old age: occupational therapy and functional illness, in *Occupational Therapy with the Elderly*. Helm, M. (Ed.) Churchill Livinstone, Edinburgh.

Blair, S.E.E. (1990) The elderly, in *Occupational Therapy and Mental Health*. Creek, J. (Ed.) Churchill Livingstone, Edinburgh.

Docherty, F. & Harley, I. (1987) Day hospitals, in *Occupational Therapy with the Elderly*. Helm, M. (Ed.) Churchill Livingstone, Edinburgh.

Harding, J. (1994) Community care, in *Knowledge to Care: A Handbook for Care Assistants*. McMahon, C.A. & Harding, J. (Eds) Blackwell Science, Oxford.

Maclean, J. (1987) Clothing, in *Occupational Therapy with the Elderly*. Helm, M. (Ed.) Churchill Livingstone, Edinburgh.

Further reading

Age Concern (1995) *Caring for Older People at Home: Staff Guidelines*. Age Concern, 82, Russia Lane, London E2 9LU.

Bender, M. (1995) An active solution for health, *Elderly Care*, Aug/Sept, **7** (4), 20.

Bluglass, R. (1983) *A Guide to the Mental Health Act 1983*, 2nd edn. Churchill Livingstone, Edinburgh.

Darby, S. & Benson, S. (Eds) (1995) *The Handbook for Community Care Assistants and Support Workers*. Hawker Publications, London.

Dennis, L. (1994) Care workers course, *Care to Make a Difference*. Alzheimer's Disease Society, London.

Duncan, I. (1987) Different types of housing and homes, in *Occupational Therapy with the Elderly*. Helm, M. (Ed.), Churchill Livingstone, Edinburgh.

Foodsense (1991) *Food Safety*. A guide from the Food Safety Directorate Ministry of Agriculture, Fisheries and Food. Available from Foodsense, London, SE99 7TT. Tel: 0181 694 8862.

Loudon, S. (1993) Positively passive, *Nursing Times.* 4 August, **89** (31), 71.

Lyall, J. (1993) Beyond bingo, *Nursing Times.* 8 September, **89** (36), 16.

Rabins, P.V. & Lucas, M.J. (1982) The impact of dementia on the family, *Journal of American Medical Association* (248), 333–335.

Ruddlesden, M. (1995) *You Can Do it! Exercises for Older People.* Hawker, London.

Smith, E.A. (1995) *Working with People With a Disabilty: Support Services at Home: Training Programme for Care Workers.* British Association for Services to the Elderly, Wales, 4th Floor, Transport House, 1 Cathedral Road, Cardiff CF1 9SD, Wales.

West, S. (1995) *Your Rights 1995–96. A Guide to Money Benefits for Older People.* 23rd edn. Age Concern England, London.

Williams, J. (1993) Rehabilitation challenge, *Nursing Times.* 4 August, **89** (31), 67.

Useful addresses

The following are able to offer help on legal and financial issues and may be worth consulting:

Benefit Enquiry Line   general advice   Tel: 0800 88 22 00
                       completing forms   Tel: 0800 44 11 44

Age Concern England
1268 London Road
London, SW16 4ER
Tel: 0181 679 8000

Citizens Advice Bureau (CAB)
You can find out where your nearest CAB is from the telephone directory or at your local library.

Law Centres Federation   Tel: 0171 387 8570

Local Social Services Office

Counsel and Care
Twyman House
16, Bonny Street
London, NW1 9PG.
Tel: 0171 485 1566

Alzheimer's Disease Society's legal advisor   Tel: 0171 306 0606

Abbeyfield Society
Abbeyfield House
53 Victoria Street
St Albans
Herts HL1 3UW

Section 4
Activities of Living

Chapter 8
Nutrition for the Older person
Jane Powell

Overview

Malnutrition is more common in older people than any other group in the population. Reasons for this include:

- Physical disability
- Mental health problems such as dementia
- Poverty
- Loneliness
- Difficulty in buying or preparing foods
- If a client has a poor diet they will be at a greater risk of many illnesses and will have a slower recovery rate.

As a carer it is very important to help your client to eat well and thereby promote good health. The information in this chapter will help you to do this.

Key words

Dietary recommendations for a healthy diet, daily nutritional targets, menu planning, monitoring food and drink, constipation, obesity, diabetes, weight loss, food hygiene, food choice and eating habits, serving food, eating environment.

What is a healthy diet for older people?

In 1992 the Department of Health issued a report titled *The Nutrition of Elderly People* (Department of Health, 1992). This report gives dietary recommendations for older people and is the basis of healthy eating advice.

The main recommendations include the following. Older people should eat a balanced and varied diet consisting of high quality nutritious foods.

Fruit and vegetables should be encouraged in order to help increase the intake of vitamin C. This is especially true for older people reliant on institutional catering where the over cooking of vegetables destroys much of the vitamin C present (Fig. 8.1).

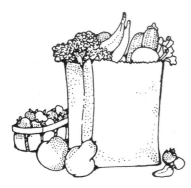

Fig. 8.1 Fruit as a source of vitamin C.

High fibre foods should be encouraged to help prevent constipation and associated problems. (Refer to the section on Constipation for list of high fibre foods.) A fluid intake of 1.5 litres of non-alcoholic fluid each day is recommended to aid the action of dietary fibre. Raw bran should be avoided as it can interfere with the absorption of calcium, iron and other minerals.

Vitamin D is made by the body when sunlight shines on the skin. Older people should be encouraged to expose some skin to sunlight regularly from May to September. If this is not possible, a vitamin D supplement should be considered.

Older people are recommended to drink 1.5 litres (2.5 pints or 8 tea cups) of fluid per day. This can be in any form but does not include alcoholic drinks. Milk is an excellent source of calcium, while fruit juice is a valuable source of vitamin C. Many older people have a reduced sense of thirst and some may be nervous to drink for fear of incontinence. Ensure that drinks are offered frequently throughout the day and encourage those clients who are hesitant to drink.

Too much fat in the diet can lead to weight gain and obesity. Certain fats are linked to an increased risk of heart disease. The dietary recommendation is that the total amount of fat in the diet should be reduced and that saturated fats in particular should be reduced. When possible, unsaturated fats should be used in place of saturated fats. Fatty/oily fish, such as mackerel, herring, tuna, etc. contain a type of fat or oil which is beneficial to the heart and should therefore be encouraged.

Saturated fats are mainly animal fats, sources include:

- Meat: beef, pork, lamb, lard, dripping, poultry fat
- Dairy products: full-fat milk, cream, cheese, butter
- Fats/oils: coconut oil palm oil unspecified vegetable oil, hard margarine

Unsaturated fats, including polyunsaturated fats, are oils from vegetables and fatty fish, sources include:

- Fatty fish: mackerel, herring, salmon, trout, tuna
- Margarines: sunflower, olive oil and other polyunsaturated margarines
- Oils: sunflower, corn, soya, olive

For frail older people or those with a poor appetite fat can be a valuable source of energy and certain vitamins. It can also help to make food more appetizing (e.g. mayonnaise in an egg sandwich). Encourage these clients to eat whatever foods they can.

Too much sugar in the diet can lead to weight gain and obesity as well as tooth decay. Sugary foods (such as sweets, sugary drinks, sweet biscuits and cakes) contain energy but little protein, vitamins or minerals. These sugary foods are not very nutritious and may reduce the appetite for more important high quality foods. The recommendation is to reduce the amount of sugar and sugary foods in the diet.

For frail, older people or those with a poor appetite, sugar and sugary foods can be useful for providing energy in a small quantity of food, and can make food more appetizing. In this situation sugar and sugary foods should be used in addition to more nourishing foods, e.g. drinking chocolate can be added to milk to make a more attractive bedtime drink.

Older people are advised to make moderate reduction in their salt intake to reduce the risk of heart disease, strokes and to help those suffering from high blood pressure. A severe reduction should only be made on medical advice. It should be noted that a low intake of salt in the diet can lead to sodium depletion and confused mental state in those taking diuretics (water tablets). Also a low salt diet tends to be bland and unappetizing. If trying to reduce the amount of salt in the diet, other forms of seasoning should be used.

Note: If your client has a poor appetite, is underweight or suffering from a chronic illness, their diet should be discussed with a senior member of the care team before trying to apply the healthy eating recommendations. It may be more appropriate for them to keep to their normal eating habits.

Are vitamins and minerals important?

A good dietary supply of vitamins and minerals is essential. If your client is eating a well-balanced diet with plenty of variety and in appropriate quantities it is likely that they are getting all the vitamins and minerals they need. However, if they have a poor diet or appetite, or if they have increased dietary needs due to illness, it may be necessary for your client to take a vitamin supplement (Table 8.1).

What is a balanced diet?

To help ensure that nutritional recommendations are met, *minimum daily nutritional targets* can be used (see Table 8.2). It must be stressed that these are the minimum amounts of food to be taken each day; the actual amounts needed for an individual will vary according to age, sex and activity levels.

Menu planning

The client should be encouraged to take an active part in planning their own menu. As a carer you can help, encourage, support and advise your

Table 8.1 Sources of important vitamins and minerals.

Vitamin B complex		
Vitamin B1 (thiamin)	Wholegrain cereals, nuts, meat, fish, pulses, yeast extract	Help in the breakdown of foods to provide energy
Vitamin B2 (riboflavin)	Liver, milk, eggs	
Nicotinic acid	Whole grain cereals, meat fish, liver pulses.	Used by the nervous system
Folid Acid and Vitamin B12	Liver, green vegetables, meat eggs, yeast extract	Blood formation, prevents anaemia
Vitamin D	Oily fish (herrings, sardines, pilchards), eggs, margarine, yoghurt, evaporated milk and breakfast cereals	Helps to keep bones healthy
Calcium	Cheese, milk, yoghurt, fish, pulses, dark green vegetables	With vitamin D it helps to keep bones and teeth healthy and strong
Vitamin C	Citrus fruits and their juices, vitamin C enriched squash, blackcurrant squash, green vegetables, potatoes	Aids iron absorption, helps body to fight infection and heals wounds
Iron	Liver, kidney, red meat	Blood formation (red blood cells, haemoglobin) prevents anaemia

client in planning their menu, but your client must have the final say in choosing the foods they wish to eat.

Try to ensure that:

(1) The client's individual food preferences and their cultural and religious needs are known and have been taken into account
(2) The nutritional recommendations have been considered
(3) Any special dietary needs have been accounted for
(4) A wide variety of foods and cooking methods have been used
(5) A sufficient variety of colour, taste and texture has been included in the meals
(6) The food items on the menu are readily available
(7) The right food storage and cooking equipment and facilities are available
(8) The meal is within the budget of the client or catering department
(9) The meal is served at the appropriate time for the client
(10) The cooking practices are within the current food hygiene regulations (Foodsense, 1992)

Table 8.2 Daily nutritional targets.

Food	Quality	Comments
Milk	300–600 ml per day	Use on cereals, in puddings and drinks, yoghurt or cheese can be a useful source of calcium, as are fish, whose bones are eaten
	Two portions	
Meat Fish	60–90 g } cooked 120–150 g } weights	Red meats, corned beef are useful sources of iron; oily fish provide vitamin D
Cheese	60 g	
Eggs	2	
Pulses (beans and peas)	60 g (dried weight)	Use pulses in soups, casseroles or salads
Bread, breakfast cereal, pasta, rice, potatoes	At least one portion at each meal	Use jacket potatoes, wholemeal bread and pasta and brown rice to increase the fibre content
Vegetables: fresh or frozen, salad	Two portions per day	These provide fibre, vitamins and minerals
Fruit; fresh, stewed, tinned or dried, Fruit juices	One portion per day	Try to include citrus fruit two or three times each week
Fluids	At *least* eight cups of fluid per day	For example, water, squash, fruit juice, milk, tea, coffee: this helps to prevent constipation and maintain health

Remember that it is essential that a client's own food preferences and needs are recognised and are respected.

Monitoring food and drink

If you are requested to monitor a client's food and drink intake it must be done accurately as the information recorded will be used to assess the client's nutritional intake. You may be asked to monitor a client's food and drink intake in order to:

■ Check that the client is eating the correct quantity and type of food
■ Check the client is drinking the right quantity of fluids

Table 8.3 Food record chart.

NAME *Emma Smith*	
DATE *18 January*	Type and Quantity of food and drink
Breakfast	2 slices wholemeal toast with butter and marmalade Small glass of orange juice 2 mugs coffee with milk
Mid-morning	Mug of tea with milk 1 wholemeal biscuit
Lunch	Chicken sandwich (2 slices of wholemeal) with tomato and mayonnaise 1 pot of fruit yoghurt and 1 banana Large glass of fruit squash
Mid-afternoon	Mug of tea with milk
Supper	Grilled plaice and parsley sauce 2 medium boiled potatoes, 2 tablespoonfuls of peas Matchbox size piece of cheese and 2 cheese biscuits Large glass of water
Bedtime	Mug of hot milk
Daily foods	300 ml of milk for drinks

A food record chart can be used to monitor a client's food and drink (Table 8.3). When using this, describe the food and the quantity eaten as accurately as possible. For instance a traditional Sunday roast lunch could be recorded as:

2 slices roast beef and gravy
3 small roast potatoes
2 tablespoonful of peas
1 tablespoonful of carrots
small bowl of rice pudding
small orange juice
2 cups of tea and two teaspoonfuls of sugar

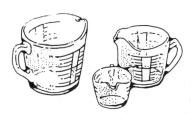

Fig. 8.2 Measuring fluids.

Household measures e.g. small bowl, teacup and mug etc. are often accurate enough, but occasionally you may need to measure food and drink more accurately, e.g. 100 ml orange juice, 50 g roast beef, 150 g rice pudding. Remember to only record the amount of food and drink eaten rather than the amount which was served (Fig 8.2).

If any foods are missed off the food chart or the amount recorded is inaccurate the health care team may assume that the client is not eating enough. This could result in the client being prescribed extra nutrients by their doctor in the form of supplementary drinks or vitamin tablets when they do not need them. Alternatively, if the carer records that the client is eating and drinking more that they actually are, it may be assumed by the care team that the client is eating well, when they may be at risk of losing weight or developing nutritional deficiencies.

If a client in not meeting their daily nutritional targets, or if you are worried about their diet it is important to notify the appropriate member of the care team as soon as possible.

Activity 8.1 ■

 Draw up your own food record chart and use this to record the amount of food and drink consumed by your client in one day. Remember to explain to your client why you are doing this. Then compare them with the recommendations for healthy eating.

■ ■

Special dietary needs

Some clients have special dietary requirements that need to be considered. In this section we will look at some of the more common therapeutic diets, religious and cultural factors affecting food choice and diets based on personal ethics and beliefs.

Therapeutic diets

More detailed information on therapeutic diets or advice for an individual client may be obtained from the nutrition and dietetic department at your local hospital or community offices. If a client needs a therapeutic diet written information and details should be included in their plan of care.

Constipation and the high fibre diet

Constipation is a common problem for the older person. It can cause a feeling of fullness, nausea, and general distress and often leads to a reduced appetite. A high fibre diet can help to prevent constipation and diverticular disease (stretching of the colon forming pouches, a result of long-standing constipation) and can help to relieve pain associated with haemorrhoids. When dietary fibre is eaten it absorbs water and softens the stools, making them easier to pass. It is therefore very important for the client to drink plenty of fluids during the day, at least 1.5 litres or eight cups, if they are eating high fibre foods.

Good sources of dietary fibre include

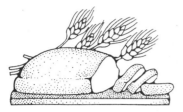

Fig. 8.3 Wholemeal bread as a source of fibre.

- Wholemeal or high bran breads (Fig. 8.3)
- Wholegrain or bran enriched breakfast cereals, e.g. Allbran, Branflakes, Weetabix, Shredded Wheat
- Foods made with wholemeal flour
- Fruits of all kinds, especially if the skin is eaten; dried fruit, prunes apricots and bananas are particularly good
- Vegetables of all kinds especially peas, beans and lentils
- Wholemeal pasta, brown rice.

It is very common for the client to experience some degree of flatulence or wind when starting to eat high fibre foods. Try to introduce high fibre foods slowly and reassure your client that the problem will soon pass.

Note: raw bran should not be given to older people as it interferes with the absorption of iron, calcium and other minerals.

Obesity and the weight reducing diet

In younger adults obesity can lead to disorders such as diabetes, high blood pressure, stroke and coronary heart disease. In older people over 75 years of age this relationship is less clearly defined, however obesity does aggravate arthritis and increases mobility problems.

Weight gain occurs when more food is eaten than the body needs, the extra calories from the food is then stored as body fat. To lose this body fat the client must eat less than the body needs, so that the fat stores are used up. It is however, still important for the client to have a good balanced diet containing the essential vitamins, minerals, protein and dietary fibre.

The following guidelines should be used for a sensible weight reducing diet:

(1) Encourage three meals a day: breakfast, lunch and supper.
(2) Between-meal snacks should be avoided
(3) Fried and fatty foods should be avoided
(4) Sweet and sugary foods should be avoided
(5) Artificial sweeteners and low calorie drinks can be used; but diabetic foods and slimming aids are not advised
(6) Fruit should be encouraged in place of puddings
(7) Encourage a good intake of high fibre foods to help satisfy the appetite
(8) All alcoholic drinks should be avoided
(9) Weight should be lost slowly and consistently 250–500 g ($\frac{1}{2}$–1 lb) a week is ideal for the older person.
(10) When possible exercise should be taken within the individual's own ability

Clients needing to lose weight for medical reasons should have a personal diet sheet preferably from a dietitian.

Weight reduction for an older person may be particularly difficult as they are often unable to exercise and may only require a relatively small quantity of food each day. To lose weight they will need to reduce this quantity still further. If a reducing diet is followed for a long period of time the client may be at risk of developing nutritional deficiencies. It is very important to monitor your client's diet carefully and encourage them to eat the correct amount from each of the five food groups in Table 8.2.

Before an older person starts a weight reducing diet, it is important to clarify why they are doing it. Think about the length of time it will take for them to reach their target weight and the dietary restrictions they will need to keep to. When weighing up the pros and cons you may find that a client's quality of life is greater following their normal eating habits and maintaining their present weight than when following a restrictive diet and losing weight. It should be the client's choice as to whether or not to follow a weight reducing diet. If they choose to do so, a senior member of the care team should be involved in monitoring their progress. Carers or other members of the team must offer plenty of support and encouragement for the duration of the diet.

Note: the decision to reduce the amount of food provided for the client should never be made by the carer or the person serving the food. It should first be discussed by the whole team including the client. Random restriction of food can have a harmful effect on the client's health.

Activity 8.2 ■■■■■■■■■■■■■■■■■■■■■■■■■■■■

 If a client wanted to reduce weight from 79.5 kg to 76.3 kg (12 stone 7 lbs to 12 stone), how long would to take if they lost an average 250 g (1/2 lb) per week. Write a menu for one day using the weight reducing guidelines and daily nutritional targets.

■■■■■■■■■■■■■■■■■■■■■■■■■■■■■■

Diabetes and the diabetic diet

Diabetes is a disorder in which the body is unable to control the amount of sugar (i.e. glucose) in the blood. It is essential to have the right amount of sugar in the blood, if the body is to function properly.

What happens normally?

Sugar is absorbed from the food in the gut into the bloodstream. For the body to use this sugar, the pancreas (a gland situated behind the stomach in the abdomen) produces a hormone called insulin. Insulin allows the sugar in the blood to pass into the cells and tissues of the body where it can be used as energy.

What happens when a person has diabetes?

Diabetes is a condition where the pancreas is unable to produce enough insulin to allow the sugar to move from the blood into the tissues. The sugar is therefore trapped in the blood and, unless treated its level will rise uncontrollably.

When the blood sugar level is too high, small amounts of sugar overflow into the urine. This can lead to problems:

- Sugar will draw water into the urine, making the diabetic person want to pass water frequently through the day and night.
- As this extra water is lost the body becomes dehydrated, causing the person to become extremely thirsty.
- Sugar in the urine is an excellent food for bacteria and can lead to urinary infection.

There are also more serious side-effects to diabetes. The likelihood of suffering these is increased if the client does not follow the correct diabetic treatment.

Treatment

- Diet alone
- Diet and insulin injections
- Diet and tablets

Whatever the form of treatment it is important to remember that the client will always need to follow a diabetic diet. Clients with diabetes should have their own personal dietary advice from a dietitian, diabetic nurse or doctor. It is important that your client's diabetic control is regularly reviewed as treatment often needs to be changed as people become older.

Dietary guidelines

The general dietary guidelines for clients with diabetes are:

(1) Eat regular meals containing starchy foods (e.g. bread, potato, pasta, rice, chapatis)
(2) Do not miss meals
(3) If recommended by a dietitian, diabetes nurse or doctor it may be necessary to take regular between-meal snacks
(4) Avoid sweet and sugary food and drink
(5) If overweight try to lose the extra weight
(6) Try to eat a wholemeal or high fibre food with each meal
(7) Do not use diabetic products as they are expensive, not low calorie and some contain a sweetener called sorbital which can cause diarrhoea. Diabetic squash and jams or marmalade may be taken

(8)   Avoid fat and fatty food (especially if the client is overweight)
(9)   Alcohol may be taken in moderation but not on an empty stomach
(10)   Sweet alcoholic drinks should be avoided

These are only general guidelines and you will find that individual dietary advice may vary slightly.

A diabetic diet can sometimes appear off-putting especially if the client needs to make changes to their eating habits. Occasionally, this can result in the client eating very little and losing their appetite. If this happens, check they are not losing weight and notify a senior member of the care team.

Hypoglycaemia (low blood sugar)

Older people who are taking insulin or certain diabetic tablets may be affected by hypoglycaemic attacks (often called a *hypo*). This is when the blood sugar becomes too low. Early warning signs vary from person to person and include shaking, trembling, confusion, sweating, tingling sensations, palpitations and becoming absent-minded or argumentative. Diabetic persons usually recognize their own symptoms.

Hypoglycaemia can arise if a client taking insulin or certain diabetic drugs:

- Misses or delays a meal or snack
- Takes strenuous exercise over and above their usual level of exercise
- Does not eat enough starchy foods
- Takes more insulin than is needed by the body
- Takes too much alcohol

How should hypoglycaemia be treated?

Hypoglycaemia must be treated immediately, if not your client could lose consciousness. If your client has any of the symptoms already mentioned, try to get them to take a small amount of sugary food, for example:

- 1 egg-cupful of Lucozade (50 ml)
- 3 Dextrol tablets
- 150 ml (3/4 cup) of ordinary lemonade

- 2 lumps/teaspoonful of sugar
- 100 ml (1/2 cup) of ordinary Coke

This should make them feel better within a few minutes, after which they should have:

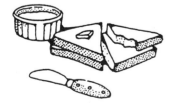

either 1 cup of milk and a biscuit
or 2 digestive biscuits
or 2 slices of bread as a sandwich (Fig. 8.4)

Fig. 8.4 A sandwich.

Alternatively if it is time for their next meal they should eat it straight away. If your client frequently suffers from hypos their doctor should be notified.

Note: if your client has lost consciousness do not attempt to give them a drink or put food in their mouth as this will cause them to choke. Find out what the policy is in your workplace for treating an unconscious hypo-glycaemic client.

What if a diabetic becomes ill?

If a diabetic client, taking insulin or diabetic tablets, becomes ill it is very important that they do not stop taking their medication. This is because illness (e.g. influenza, diarrhoea, colds) will cause a natural rise in blood sugar. Non-diabetic people can cope with this but people with diabetes must continue to take their medication in order to control it. It is important that your client takes regular meals and snacks. If they do not feel like a full meal, encourage them to take frequent snacks through the day, such as soup and bread, yoghurt, sandwiches.

Weight loss and poor appetite

Weight loss occurs when a client has a poor appetite, when food intake is reduced or when illness causes an increased energy requirement, i.e. when more energy is used by the body than is being eaten in the diet. If a client is poorly nourished they should be encouraged to take a high energy, high protein diet in order to meet their nutritional needs.

Appetite can be increased by encouraging small, frequent meals regularly throughout the day and by offering foods which are enjoyable and attractively presented. People need plenty of encouragement to eat if they have a poor appetite but with perseverance their appetite should improve.

High protein foods such as meat, fish, eggs, cheese and milk should be encouraged. Try offering milky drinks instead of tea, coffee or squash. Milk can be made more nutritious by adding two tablespoonfuls of milk powder to one pint of whole milk. This fortified milk can be used for drinks, cereals and in cooking, etc.

Avoid giving large quantities of food as this can often be a turn-off for a client with a poor appetite.

Dietary supplements are a useful way of adding extra nourishment to the diet. They are products which contain a concentrated source of nourishment in a relatively small quantity. They are usually in the form of drinks and can be bought from chemists or obtained on a prescription for certain medical conditions. Examples include Build-up, Complan, and Vitafood (available from a chemist) and Fortisip, Fresubin and Ensure (available on prescription only). If your client has been advised to take a dietary supplement encourage them to take it regularly as advised by their doctor or dietitian.

It should be remembered that a reduction in body weight is only one indicator of a poor diet and only relates to energy intake. Deficiencies of other nutriments can occur while body weight remains constant. Skin changes, poor wound healing, anaemia and self-neglect may be indicators of poor diet. If you feel that your client is at risk of developing nutritional deficiencies, notify the care team, client's doctor or dietitian.

Religious and cultural factors affecting food choice

In many religions there are rules or conventions about food. Your client may have strong views on which food they will not eat depending on their degree of orthodoxy. Clarify this with each client and ensure their rules are adhered to. McMahon & Harding (1994) has more detailed information about this.

People from different cultures may prefer to eat their own traditional foods instead of a Western diet. Foods from different cultures are widely available; try to make yourself familiar with these foods and ensure your client has access to them whenever possible.

Diets based on personal ethics and beliefs

Many people choose to eat a diet based on personal ethics or beliefs. Examples of this include vegetarian or vegan diets or the use of free-range or organic produce.

If you are providing food for a vegetarian or vegan it is important to know how to provide a healthy balanced diet without the use of animal products. There are many vegetarian and vegan recipe books available. Choose one which contains as explanation of the principles of a balanced diet.

It is more difficult to provide food for a client wishing to eat organic or free-range foods. Find out if these foods are available in local shops or whether a local supplier can be found; the client's relatives may be an additional source of information. If you are unable to provide the food your client wishes to eat, talk to your client to find out if they are willing to accept a compromise.

Swallowing and swallowing difficulties

On average a person will swallow over 600 times in a 24 hour period. We not only swallow when we eat or drink, but also swallow saliva constantly through the day and night. Swallowing is a very complex procedure, the muscles of the mouth and face must be in full working order to swallow properly and easily.

Normal swallowing can be divided into three stages;

(1)   The mouth (oral stage)
(2)   The throat (pharyngeal stage)
(3)   The tube leading to the stomach (oesophageal stage)

(see *Knowledge to Care* (1994) Chapter 9, Nutrition)

Swallowing difficulties (dysphasia) can be caused by a variety of disorders including stroke, Parkinson's disease, multiple sclerosis and head injury.

Any degree of dysphasia can be uncomfortable and frightening for the client. There are ways of helping dysphagic clients to swallow and it is vitally important to follow any specific guidelines or plan of care your client may have. If you ignore these guidelines you will be putting your client at risk of choking or developing a chest infection.

If your client suffers from dysphasia it is likely to affect their ability and desire to eat and drink. You may need to prepare food of a specific consistency or you may need to thicken all their drinks so they are easier to swallow. Each client should be separately assessed and advice given for their individual needs. Your local speech and language therapist can give specific advice regarding individual needs. Care must be taken to ensure the client is sitting in an upright position to eat and the carer should watch for any signs of choking while they are eating or drinking.

Swallowing and the care required for clients with swallowing difficulties is covered in more detail in *Knowledge to Care* (1994)

Activity 8.3 ■

 Liquidized food can look very unappetizing. Draw up a breakfast and lunch menu for a client requiring liquidized food. Think of five ways to help make the meal look attractive.

■ ■

Food hygiene

There are four groups of people who are most at risk from food poisoning. These are babies and young children, pregnant women, older people and those who are ill. For people in these groups food poisoning can cause severe illness and occasionally death. The topic 'Food Hygiene' not only covers the storage of food, preparation and cooking of food, but also buying food and personal hygiene of those in contact with food. (Foodsense, 1992)

Food poisoning is an illness caused by food or drink contaminated by disease causing bacteria, viruses or chemicals. Bacteria are the most common cause of food poisoning.

Activity 8.4 ■

  Can you list the symptoms of food poisoning?

■ ■

The time between eating infected foods and the onset of symptoms can be from one hour to three days, but it is usually between 12 and 36 hours. The symptoms can last from six hours to eight days, but usually last one to three days. The symptoms of food poisoning are:

- Abdominal pain or cramps
- Diarrhoea
- Nausea, vomiting
- Fever

If you suspect your client is suffering from food poisoning notify a senior member of the care team as soon as possible. Encourage your client to drink plenty of fluids to prevent dehydration.

All foods contain a low level of bacteria. When certain bacteria multiply to reach high levels, food poisoning occurs. For bacteria to multiply they require four conditions: *food to grow on, moisture, warmth, time.*

If one of these is not present the bacteria will only multiply slowly. For example, dried foods such as dried milk keep for a long time because they contain little water. Of the above four conditions the easiest to regulate is temperature. At temperatures below 5°C food poisoning bacteria stop multiplying, but are not killed. At temperatures above 63°C bacteria start to die. The range of temperatures between 10–63°C is called the 'danger zone' in which bacteria can multiply rapidly and cause food poisoning. This is why perishable foods should be kept in a refrigerator or freezer and all cooked foods should be heated until they reach a temperate above 70°C and served piping hot not lukewarm. Food poisoning bacteria grow best at 37°C (i.e. body temperature), it is therefore very important that they are not eaten in large quantities.

Buying foods

You cannot tell how safe food is by its look or smell.

Perishable foods are labelled with 'use by' or 'sell by' dates. Do not use food beyond its 'use by' date. It is illegal for shops to sell foods beyond the 'sell by' date, do not be tempted to buy old food at reduced prices.

Avoid buying food from shops which are storing food badly. For instance you may find defrosted foods in the freezer section or overstocked refrigerators which do not chill food properly.

Do not buy food if the packaging is damaged. Bacteria can be transmitted from raw food onto cooked food. When buying food from a delicatessen check that the sales person is not handling raw food and cooked food without washing their hands or changing their gloves.

Carefully wrap raw meat, poultry or fish before packing it in to your shopping bag. This will prevent juices from raw foods dripping onto cooked foods. Pack chilled or frozen foods together to try to keep cool on the journey home. If possible use an insulated container such as a 'cool bag/box to transport them.

Do not keep chilled or frozen foods at room temperature for any longer that necessary, as rises in temperature will encourage bacteria to multiply. Put them into a refrigerator or freezer as soon as possible.

Food storage

Use a refrigerator thermometer to check that the refrigerator is kept at 5°C, or lower; this will prevent bacteria multiplying.

Make sure the refrigerator door shuts properly, defrost it regularly and keep it clean. Do not leave the refrigerator door open any longer than absolutely necessary.

Keep cooked foods covered and place them on the top shelf of the refrigerator. Always keep raw or defrosting meat, poultry or fish covered in a container to catch the drips. This will prevent raw foods dripping onto cooked foods thereby contaminating them with bacteria. Carefully follow any storage instructions on foods, e.g. refrigerate after opening.

Defrost the freezer regularly so that it works efficiently. When cleaning the freezer, ensure that any frozen foods are kept frozen either in a neighbour's freezer, in a cool box or wrapped in newspaper. Do not refreeze any food which has defrosted, cook it straight away.

Check that food is not kept beyond its 'use by' date. This includes dry products such as flour and custard powder. Ensure that new foods are put to the back of the cupboard and older foods used first.

Food preparation

Always wash your hands thoroughly before cooking or touching foods. Dry them on a clean handtowel as bacteria can be transferred from your hands, onto the teatowel and the onto the clean dishes.

Keep work surfaces clean. Disinfect food preparation areas regularly, especially after preparing raw meat, poultry or fish on work surfaces.

Disinfect kitchen cloths regularly or use disposable cloths and sponges which are regularly renewed.

Do not use the same cooking utensils for preparing raw and cooked foods without washing them first. For example, if a kitchen knife is used to cut raw chicken and then a slice of cheese this can cause food poisoning.

Use clean hot water and detergent for washing up. Never use a dirty teatowel to dry the dishes, it is preferable to let them drip dry.

Keep the kitchen clean at all times. Wipe up all food spills immediately and keep the floor clean. This will help to prevent the infestation of flies, ants, cockroaches and mice.

Cooking food

Ensure that frozen meat and poultry is thoroughly defrosted before cooking. This should be done in the refrigerator or microwave, but never at room temperature as this will encourage bacteria to grow.

Follow cooking instructions on food labels carefully. It is not safe to put food into a cold oven before cooking. Cook food until it is piping hot, above 70°C. Make sure the food is cooked right through.

Eggs should be cooked thoroughly in order to kill any food bacteria (Salmonella) which may be present. Never give raw eggs in any form to vulnerable people (including older people). Eggs should be hard boiled, omelettes well cooked and home made mayonnaise or mousse containing raw egg should be avoided.

If keeping cooked food, do not put it into the refrigerator while still hot, keeping it covered, cool it first in a cool part of the kitchen. If possible within an hour of cooking.

Do not reheat cooked foods more than once.

Catering policies

In 1990 the Government issued the Food Safety Act which set out hygiene regulations for any premises producing food, but does not apply to the client's own home.

Individual care homes and hospitals have developed their own food policies based on the 1990 Food Safety Act. It is essential that you follow the food policy regulation in your own work place.

Activity 8.5   ■

 Read your own organization's food handling policy.

■ ■

Factors affecting food choice and eating habits

As we have already seen there are many reasons why people choose to eat certain foods. Your client may follow dietary restrictions for medical or religious reasons or they may wish to choose foods which they feel will give them a healthy balanced diet.

When first getting to know your client make sure you are aware of any issues which may affect their food choice and eating habits. Your client will prefer certain foods and most people have favourite foods or meals. Try to make a list of your clients food preferences, but remember that it will need to be updated on a regular basis.

There are many factors affecting food and drink choice, physical and mental factors play a large part and include;

- Poor dentition and chewing difficulties
- Swallowing difficulties
- Deterioration of taste and smell
- Communication difficulties
- Poor vision

- Physical disability
- Breathing difficulty
- Constipation and incontinence
- Side-effects of drugs
- Mental health problems

Environmental and social factors can also affect food choice and eating habits and are discussed in the next section.

If your client needs to follow a special diet you should try to support, encourage and help them to do so but ultimately you must respect your client's own choice of food and drink. If they are not happy with the food being offered to them you must provide a suitable alternative. If your client has a very poor appetite or extreme food preferences it can be difficult to provide a meal which they feel able to eat. In this situation make sure that a senior member for the care team is aware of the problem. It may be necessary to monitor the client's food and drink intake to assess whether they are eating enough.

Issues outside the client's control can also affect the type of food available to them. If the carer is providing food in the client's home the following points can influence which type of foods are prepared. They include;

- Money available to spend on food
- Distance to the shops and the time allocated to do the shopping
- Type of shops nearby (do they sell the foods your client likes?)
- Food storage facilities (refrigerator, freezer, cupboards)
- Cooking facilities and cooking equipment (cooker, microwave, measuring jug, etc.)
- Time allocated to cook, serve and clear away meals

When food is being provided by an outside source (meals on wheels, catering department in a hospital or care home) there is usually only a limited choice of food available. This choice must be appropriate to the client group being catered for. Most types of institutional catering keep to a preset menu, although small establishments may cater according to individual requests. Catering departments have a limited budget and must provide a suitable menu within these limitations. They should also provide therapeutic diets and cater for religious food preferences. Ideally all catering departments should carry out regular surveys to ensure that the menu provided is appropriate and is liked by the clients.

Activity 8.6 ■■■■■■■■■■■■■■■■■■■■■■■■■■■■■■

Write a short questionnaire to find out what your clients think about the food provided for them. Find out if therapeutic diets are available at meal times and also whether religious food preferences are catered for.

■■■■■■■■■■■■■■■■■■■■■■■■■■■■■■■■■■

Serving food and the eating environment

Making meals a pleasant experience can go a long way towards improving a client's diet. If little thought or effort is put into preparing and serving a client's meal, the client is likely to lose interest in food, let their appetite dwindle and consequently be at risk of malnutrition (Fig. 8.5). Just think, if every meal was served luke warm, the vegetables overcooked and you were sitting with people you did not know, would you look forward to the next meal?

Fig. 8.5 Serving food.

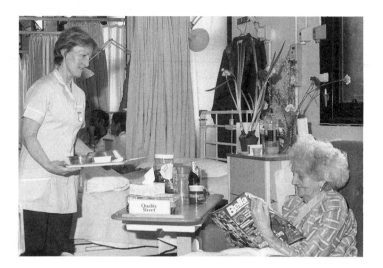

As a carer you should be aware of the issues involved in preparing the eating environment and serving food so that your client can get the most out of the food available to them. The following list shows some of the ways meal times can be made more pleasant;

- Encourage clients to do as much as possible for themselves.
- Serve food at a time preferred by the client.
- Allow clients to eat at their own pace. Never hurry them to finish.
- When necessary, help your client to move to the area they wish to eat in.
- Help your client to obtain a safe comfortable position for eating and drinking.
- Ask your client if they wish to go to the toilet and wash their hands before and after eating, when necessary help them to achieve this.
- If necessary help your client to wipe away excess food from their face, hands and clothing during and after a meal. Do this in a way which does not cause them to lose their dignity.
- If your client would like to be provided with protection for their clothes such as an apron or serviette, help them to position it so that they do not lose their dignity, and their food intake is not restricted.

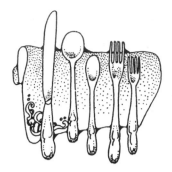

Fig. 8.6 Cutlery and napkin.

- When possible, clients should have freedom about where and with whom they sit.
- Try to ensure that the environment for eating is pleasant and accommodates the wishes of the client.
- When possible, use tablecloths, serviettes, and attractive crockery and cutlery (Fig. 8.6).
- Remove unnecessary items from the area the client wishes to eat in, e.g. Zimmer frames, commodes, nursing/medical notes, urine bottles, etc.
- Meal times may be the highlight of the day for many clients. Try to make meal times an enjoyable social occasion.
- The choice of food available should be well displayed or explained clearly to your client.
- Ensure that personal taste preferences are known and catered for.
- Encourage clients to choose the most suitable and appropriate options, and when asked, explain the reasons for this. Give the final say in choosing the food *they* wish to eat.
- If your client dislikes the food offered, provide an alternative.
- Serve food in sensible portion sizes or as the client needs or wishes.
- Try to ensure that the presentation, consistency and temperature of the food and drink served are as the client needs or wishes.
- Provide a range of condiments which are in easy reach of your client, e.g. salt, pepper, pickles, mustard, horseradish, relish, etc.
- When possible, encourage your client to serve themselves or, if eating in a communal setting to serve others.
- If possible, food should be served as it would be in an individual's home, i.e. serving dishes placed on the table, meat carved at the table etc.
- Ensure food is placed within easy reach of the client.
- Encourage social contact at meal times between clients or carer and client.
- Help your client to eat in a socially acceptable manner.
- In a communal setting provide appropriate seating arrangements for clients with antisocial eating habits.
- Having to be fed often feels undignified. Respect your client's dignity and help them to do as much as possible for themselves.
- Ensure that any eating or drinking aids are used properly.
- Avoid interrupting client during meal times.
- Clear up well after a meal and dispose of any left-over food safely.
- Ensure that the client is offered and has easy access to suitable and enjoyable food and drink between meals.
- Follow the current food hygiene regulations whenever dealing with food and drink.

Activity 8.6 ■

Tick those points in the above list which you feel you do already and put a cross against the ones you need to pay more attention to.

Of the points you have crossed, choose the five which you think are the most important. Think of how you can incorporate these into your work.

■ ■

Summary

In this chapter we have looked at a number of issues related to nutrition. An understanding of healthy eating and special dietary needs is important, but unless the food is appetizing and served in the right environment it will not be eaten in appropriate quantities to have optimum effect. Only food which is eaten will nourish the client.

Eating is a fundamental part of our lives. A carer's positive attitude to help clients with eating and drinking will increase the likelihood of the client achieving a good nutritional intake.

References

Department of Health (1992) *The Nutrition of Elderly People* (report on Health and Social Subjects, 43). HMSO, London.

Foodsense (1992) *The Food Safety Act 1991 and You. A Guide for the Food Industry.* HMSO Publications PBO 351. Available from Foodsense, London SE99 7TT (Tel 0645 556000).

McMahon, C. & Harding, J. (Eds) (1994) *Knowledge to Care.* Blackwell Science, Oxford.

Further reading

Andrews, C. (1993) Mixed meals: ileostomy diet. *Nursing Times*, 27 October, **89** (66), 43.

Archibald, B. *et al.* (1994) *Food and Nutrition in the Care of People with Dementia.* Available from Dementia Services, University of Stirling, FK9 4LA, Scotland.

Beadle, L. (1995) The management of dysphagia in stroke (to avoid malnutrition). *Nursing Standard*, 4 January, **9** (15), 37.

Blackshaw, D. & Gates, J. (1993) Handling food safely. *Elderly Care*, March/April **5** (2), 20.

Campbell, J. (1993) The mechanics of eating and drinking. *Nursing Times*, 21 May, **89** (21), 32.

Charalambous, L. (1993) A healthy approach. *Nursing Times*, 19 May, **89** (20), 59.

Department of Health (1991) *Dietary Reference Values for Food and Energy*

Nutrients for the United Kingdom. (Report of Health and Social Subjects, 41.) HMSO, London.

Dietetic Standards of Care for the Older Adult in Hospital (1993). Published by the Nutrition Advisory Group for Elderly People. Available from the British Diabetic Association.

Eating Through the 90s (1989) Published by the Nutrition Advisory Group for Elderly People. Available from the British Diabetic Association.

Eating Well for Older People (1995) Report of an expert working group. The Caroline Walker Trust.

Fairbrother, M. (1993) What can you eat? *Nursing Times*, 7 April, **89** (14), 63.

Flowers, M. (1993) Survival rations. *Nursing Times*, 30 June, **89** (11), 61.

Holmes, S. (1993) Force of habits. *Nursing Times*, 1 September **89** (35), 48.

Marshall, D. (1995) Eat your greens: the Scottish consumer's perspective on fruit and vegetables. *Health Education Journal*, June, **54** (2), 186.

Ministry of Agriculture, Fisheries and Food (1991) *Food Safety.* Available from Foodsense, London SE99 7TP (Tel 0645 556000).

Ministry of Agriculture, Fisheries and Food (1993) *Healthy Eating for Older People.* Available from Foodsense, London SE99 7TP (Tel 0645 556000).

Wynn, M. (1993) Catering concerns, *Nursing Times*, 19 May, **89** (11), 26.

Useful addresses

The British Dietetic Association
7th Floor Elizabeth House
22 Suffolk Street
Queensway
Birmingham B1 1LS
Tel 0121 643 5483

The British Diabetic Association
10 Queen Anne Street
London W1M 0BD
Tel: 0171 323 1531

College of Speech and Language
  Therapists
Bath Place
Rivington Street
London EC2A BDR
Tel: 0171 613 3855

Chapter 9

Meeting Elimination Needs
Angela Arnold

Overview

This chapter will consider normal elimination and factors that can influence elimination, which are physical, psychological, sociocultural, environmental and economic.

The following points concerning elimination will be discussed.

- Problems with elimination
- Constipation
- Incontinence
- Ways to assist the client are described
- Other members of the health care team are described
- The different aids and equipment that are suggested by them to assist with elimination are outlined
- Specimen collection and testing of urine and faeces is described as well as the recording of this output.

Key words

Normal elimination and abnormalities, privacy, specimen collection, hygiene, incontinence.

Normal elimination

'Eliminate ... to remove, to get rid of waste products.' Elimination is an activity of living which all individuals perform throughout their lives. It consists of urinary elimination, in which the urinary system produces and expels urine, and the faecal elimination where the colon produces and excretes faeces.

Normal elimination is therefore the body's way of removing waste products and toxic substances through the digestive and genito-urinary system, after the body has extracted the goodness from the food and drink the person has consumed (Figs 9.1 and 9.2).

During the day, the individual will go to the toilet in order to pass urine, at varying intervals, depending on their work and social activities. Most people however, pass urine when they wake, before or after meals and

Fig. 9.1 Urinary system.

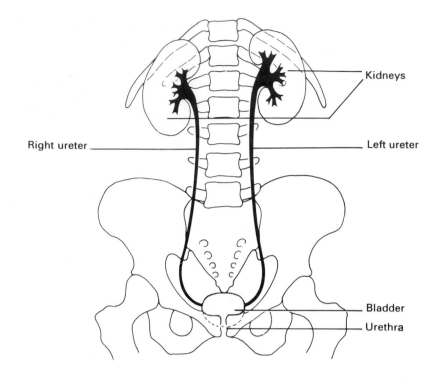

Fig. 9.2 Digestive system.

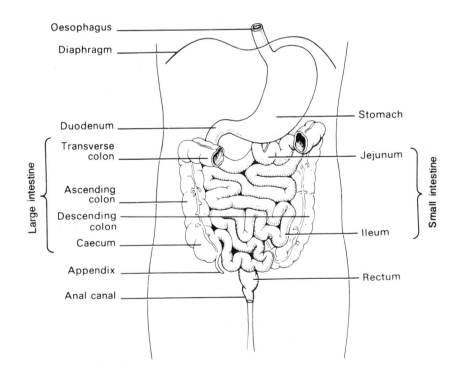

before going to bed. This may vary from five to seven times a day in the normal bladder, but can be more frequent depending on bladder capacity and control. This control is possible because messages from the brain can be blocked by conscious (voluntary) control – called inhibition. This control can help in most cases to prevent the bladder from being squeezed to pass urine. However, many older people may need assistance to use the toilet more regularly, depending on their bladder control.

Skills needed

Activity 9.1 ■

What skills do you check the older person needs to have control of when passing urine?

■ ■

The client needs to be able to start to pass urine at a suitable time, to be able to postpone it when necessary, and to anticipate the need to urinate well in advance if they are going on a long journey or if a toilet is not going to be easily accessible.

The client also needs to start passing urine when the bladder is partly full and to be able to control and interrupt the flow of urine when necessary (i.e. if disturbed). They must be able to postpone bladder emptying during sleep and respond by waking up in time when the bladder is full.

The client must also be able to identify places and circumstances where it is socially acceptable to pass urine and to be able to use the facilities provided, i.e. wash their hands afterwards.

These may once have been learnt and now the client, due to either an illness or an injury, no longer has all these skills. The cause may be reversible and a relearning programme may be needed by some older people to assist them to gain independence.

Activity 9.2 ■

List the loss of skills you have noticed when caring for some elderly clients. Try to remember what action was taken to help assist these clients and who was involved with the care planning?

■ ■

With a loss of skills, the cause needs to be investigated and in some cases treated by medications, surgery, aids, physiotherapy, individualized bladder training or toileting programmes.

Do you know?

'No society can call itself civilised if it treats its older generation with a lack of consideration, but consideration requires understanding and everyone needs to know about the process of ageing and the difficulties it may bring. Ultimately the quality of life of elderly people, especially the very old and frail, rests on the attitudes and perceptions of those younger than themselves.' (DHSS, 1981)

Normal ageing

Normal ageing slows down all body functions, including that of the digestive and genito-urinary tract and these systems may need to be investigated as well as the other systems of the body.

Thirst decreases with age and in many cases, the older person may not drink enough fluid during the day for efficient elimination of urine and faeces.

The sense of taste and smell also weakens and linked with loss of teeth or badly fitting dentures, insufficient food may be consumed. If the person has a limited budget they may not eat enough variety of food including vegetables and fruit which assist in preventing constipation (refer to Chapter 8). Fading vision may make journeys to buy food or cooking food difficult, so they may rely on processed or tinned food.

The production of saliva and gastric juices is reduced. There is a slower peristalsis (a wave-like contraction and relaxation which travels along the alimentary canal pushing the contents along). This results in more water being absorbed from faeces, leading to constipation.

Bladder control

The bladder muscles may not be so efficient, their strength diminishes and the bladder capacity may reduce. Lack of oestrogen in post-menopausal women can result in non-specific urethritis (inflammation of the urethra).

The central nervous system also changes with age. This is involved with receiving and sending messages to and from the brain regarding bladder control. This may result in an increased frequency of urine with a noticeable change being the need to wake at night to pass urine. Sleep patterns change and balance and co-ordination may be affected (refer to Chapter 10, Hygiene, Comfort and Rest).

The feeling of a full bladder and bowel can be reduced and clients often feel urgency to pass urine at the same time as a feeling of elimination is felt. This may stop them planning long journey or social occasions to friends or relatives and can lead to isolation and depression.

Diseases and disabilities

As a client ages, diseases and disabilities which may have been chronic throughout their lives or may now have become acute illness affect them. Chronic illnesses such as osteoarthritis, diabetes, cardiac (heart) troubles, nerve damage causing limited or reduced feelings in bones and joints and chronic bronchitis can affect mobility. Acute illnesses or accidents such as a chest infection with breathlessness, fractured hip or strokes can affect balance, co-ordination and mobility.

Mental disorders

Mental disorders can affect the older person, for example, depression and dementia (refer to Chapter 1). These can lead to dependence on the carer in the home or in hospital and problem behaviour such as aggression can develop. It can also lead to incontinence.

Exercise

Some clients may have been inactive in the home or in hospital for long periods of time due to several of the factors above and this can result in a lack of muscle tone of the abdominal muscles. The elimination system relies on stimulation from the muscle movements in the abdomen to function effectively. It is important to encourage the client with activities and regular walks to the toilet (if the care plan states mobility to be encouraged).

Bowel problems

Long or short-term medication can cause diarrhoea and constipation. It is important that you tell the person in charge if there is any change in the bowel habits of the clients, as it may be a side-effect of the medication and the doctor will need to be informed.

On admission to the hospital or when you visit the client in the home, the client or relatives may advise you that the client has a history of taking laxatives as they feel it is important to have a bowel movement every day. You must inform the person in charge if the person has brought their own laxatives into hospital, or is taking regular laxatives at home.

Changes in the health balance

It is important to state that in healthy older people the normal pattern of elimination differs only slightly from that of the younger person. The bladder may not hold quite as much as when they were younger and there may be some residual urine left in the bladder after voiding.

A change of environment from home to hospital or a nursing home, a minor change in health with an illness such as bronchitis however can change the balance resulting in incontinence.

Activity 9.3 ■

What do you think is the most important word when assisting clients with elimination?

■ ■

Time

Always give yourself time:

- To introduce yourself and the care team
- To explain the layout of the hospital/nursing home and where the toilets are situated
- To explain the call bell system
- To assist them to use the facilities and to help them with dressing and undressing if they need assistance
- For their hygiene needs, consider religious beliefs
- To make them comfortable after they have used the facilities
- For them to tell you any problems or anxieties they may have as regards elimination

Activity 9.4 ■

Consider your thoughts, the first time you assisted someone to the toilet. Did you consider how you would feel if you were assisted with this activity of living?

■ ■

The staff are few and they are rushed,
And mostly they are kind,
They walk me, bath me, feed my frame,
But they do not feed my mind.

Deaf ears, dim eyes, imprison me,
Just memories remain;
But they are not enough, O Lord,
Please take me whence I came.

I have been – I am – grateful still
For food and warmth and light,
But now I have no dignity,
No privacy, no right.

We even have our bottoms wiped,
In full view of the ward,
I used to say 'Please screen me off'
My words were never heard.

The patients say a nurse was blamed,
For letting someone fall,
So now the screens are stored away,
So they can watch us all.

Today I soiled my pants and chair,
Is this the end for me?

The lost control – was this a sign
Of my senility.

No, it was not my fault at all,
I called the nurse for sure,
But she was too busy, said to wait,
She'd see me to the door.

(Poem by a patient in the care of the elderly ward.)
(The Voluntary Euthanasia Society, 1992)

Genito-urinary system

The kidneys filter the body's blood, receiving a large blood flow of approximately 1200 ml per minute; however, only 1 to 1.5 litres of urine are excreted each day.

Two kidneys are situated in the upper abdomen at the back of the body (posterior). They filter out the waste products from the blood producing urine containing waste and excess water from the body.

Two hollow tubes, called ureters lead from the kidneys to the bladder, which is a hollow organ with muscular walls that expand like a balloon to hold urine. The urethra leads from the bladder to the exterior to expel urine. Urine is produced continuously day and night (there is less produced at night due to the body's natural diurnal rhythm) and a steady trickle passes down the ureters to be stored in the bladder before leaving the body (Figs 9.3 and 9.4).

Fig. 9.3 Section through male pelvis.

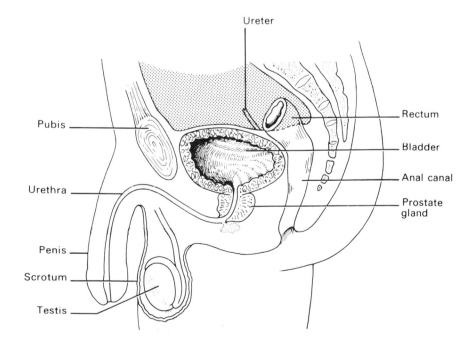

Fig. 9.4 Section through female pelvis.

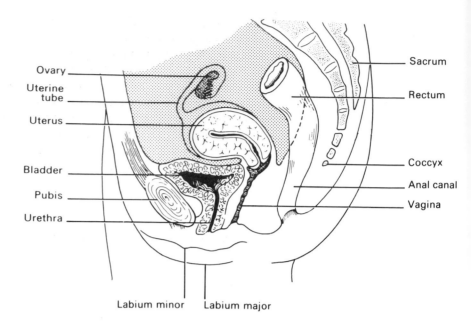

Ovary

Uterine tube

Uterus

Bladder

Pubis

Urethra

Sacrum

Rectum

Coccyx

Anal canal

Vagina

Labium minor   Labium major

Do you know?

?

In the male the urethra is 20 cms long and in the female in is about 5 cms long. Consider this in relation to urinary tract infections. In women, the distance from the outside is shorter so that micro-organisms (bacteria) only have a short distance to travel into the body and upwards through the genito-urinary system. This can lead to cystitis (inflammation of the bladder) and kidney infections. Normally the continual flow of urine down the ureters can help to reduce the chances of micro-organisms gaining access and becoming established in the body to cause these infections.

The older person in an institution has a high risk of urinary tract infections. It is suggested that the age related changes in the lower urinary tract can also reduce resistance to infection. The presence of urine retained in the bladder due to inadequate emptying when the client passes urine is another contributing factor to urinary tract infection (UTI).

The carer has an important part to play in the health care team by assisting to reduce infection by encouraging a variety of drinks through the day. As stated earlier, the clients' thirst mechanism is less effective and they may not feel the need to drink. Offer a variety of drinks, from soup, soft drinks, water and hot drinks. Ensure they are easy to reach and in containers that they can help themselves to during the day or night. The client needs to be encouraged to drink 2–3 litres a day, if the care plan states free fluids.

Urination

When approximately 100–150 mls of urine have collected in the bladder, messages are transmitted to the brain and the person becomes aware that their bladder is full and that they want to go to the toilet. If there is a convenient place and the person has time to go, they will prepare to urinate by undressing and relaxing muscles to allow urine to pass from the bladder as it contracts, and then down the urethra and out of the body. If it is inconvenient or not a suitable place, they will hold the urine in the bladder until it is convenient and the bladder will stretch to hold more urine. Adults will go to the toilet five to seven times a day and many older persons like to go every two to three hours, this may be due to an irritable bladder or the worry that they may become incontinent.

Remember that many older people feel urgency at the same time as the feeling to pass urine is felt. The average bladder can hold 350–600 ml of urine.

Activity 9.5   ■

What is the difference between frequency, urgency and leakage of urine?

■ ■

Frequency is when the bladder can only hold a small amount of urine and has to be emptied inconveniently often. *Urgency* arises when the bladder needs to be emptied in a great hurry. *Leakage* is the loss of urine, which can occur before or after a visit to the toilet.

Frequency and urgency can be caused by tea or coffee as they increase the production of urine by the kidneys (diuretic effect). A urinary tract infection, or a disturbance in the client's mental state can also have the same effect. Urgency can occur when the client is anxious or depressed, something to consider should the client change environments.

Constipation can also be a cause of frequency and urgency as the bowel presses on the bladder causing irritation. Leakage occurs when the pelvic muscles around the bladder and urethra weaken.

Observations of urine

What do you know about urine? Urine should be amber to straw coloured, nearly odourless, clear and free from mucus or sediment. It is formed by the kidneys and is the vehicle by which water and the end products of metabolism are excreted. It is 96% water, 2% salts and 2% waste products, (to include urea and creatinine). Normal urine is sterile.

If the urine is very dilute and *pale* it may be due to an excessive fluid intake, diuretic tablets (water tablets), or diabetes mellitus (diabetes). *Dark* urine may be due to concentration of urine due to a reduced fluid intake. Liver or gall bladder problems can also lead to dark urine. Medications can change the colour of urine and the presence of blood will make it smoky or frank blood may be seen (haematuria).

The urine may *smell*, if it has a sweet (acetone) smell, this must be reported and the urine tested for ketones and glucose. Infected urine can smell fishy and frank pus could be present, the urine should be tested for the presence of protein.

Observations of the client

While assisting the patient check the following:

- Did they have difficulty with mobility, undressing or dressing?
- Leakage before they reached the toilet?
- Passing urine?
- Meeting hygiene needs?
- Showing any pain or discomfort whilst passing urine?

What would you do if you noticed any problems? *Report it and record it.*

A chronic or acute urinary infection can cause a burning pain on passing urine (dysuria), loin pain, urgency or frequency. There may be blood in the urine and the client complains of a high temperature (pyrexia) and may appear confused. The urine may have an unpleasant odour.

General observations

Look   for physical and emotional changes
Listen   to the person's problems
Feel   their skin, is it hot or cold?
Smell   their urine

If there are any problems, you must save a labelled specimen of urine, report what you saw, smelt, felt or heard immediately.

If your organization allows you to record information in the care plan, record the information neatly and clearly in black ink (plus signature, date and time).

Remember, after the client has used the bedpan, commode, urinal or toilet, the contents should be checked for any abnormalities before disposal.

Do you know?

 A urinary infection (UTI) is the presence of an infective agent in the urinary tract, the most common micro-organisms are bacteria from the bowel and faeces. The most common bacteria is called Escherichia coli. (E. coli).

Follow-up

The carer may be asked to take the client's temperature and pulse, collect a specimen of urine or faeces in a sterile container.

Collecting a urine specimen
MSU (midstream specimen). This is collected in a labelled sterile container

and sent to the laboratory as soon as possible with a form written for the investigations. The first part of the urine stream is discarded as it may contain contaminating germs which will give false results.

The client needs to be advised or assisted to clean their external genitalia from front to back, with a clean cloth or swabs. (Some organizations may wish a sterile solution and swabs to be used.) They are then instructed to start passing urine – then to stop. Urine is then collected in a specimen container. When full, any excess urine is then passed down the toilet or into a bedpan. It may be difficult to collect if the client is confused or is immobile with a stroke or a fracture, and assistance may be needed. The urine may need to be collected in a sterile jug and then put into the specimen container. Do not touch the inside of the container as it will give false results. It may be helpful for a female client to sit on a toilet or bedpan facing the back, making more room to hold the jug or specimen container.

An *EMU (early morning specimen)*. The first urine passed on waking, this urine is more concentrated.

A *twenty-four hour urine collection*. This is urine collected over a 24 hour period. For example, the client is asked pass urine at 08.00 hrs and this is then discarded. All urine is collected until 08.00 hrs the following day, when the client passes urine again which is added to the collection as the final sample. It is important that if you throw away a urine sample that is part of this collection, you tell the person in charge in order that a new 24 hour collection is started, as it will give false results if urine samples are missing.

Testing of urine

This skill is first demonstrated and then practised under supervision.

Activity 9.6 ■

When do you test the urine of the client?

■ ■

- On admission
- Before an operation
- On certain medications (such as anti coagulants)
- If the client is a diabetic
- If asked to by the person in charge if an abnormality is suspected (Fig 9.5)

How to test urine

Always use a clean container that is only used for urine collection and testing. If the client is to leave a specimen for testing, it must be clearly labelled with their name, date and time. The urine should be fresh, as if it stands for a long time the contents will change. Put on gloves before starting the test.

Fig. 9.5 Testing urine.

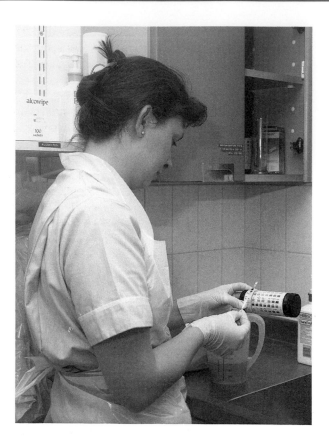

A reagent stick is used for this testing, it is taken from a bottle that should have a tightly fitting lid and the date on the bottle should not have expired.

After removing the stick, close the bottle tightly. Do not touch the end of the stick that is going in the specimen of urine. Dip the stick in the urine and ensure that the coloured squares are all covered with urine. Remove and tap lightly on the side of the container to remove any excess urine. Read the stick according to the manufacturers' instructions. Record the results and report immediately any abnormalities. Further testing of individual samples or a 24 hour collection may then be ordered to be tested in the laboratories.

What is recorded?

ph
This tells if the urine is acid or alkaline. It varies between 4.5 and 8.0, 7.0 is neutral, above 7.0 is alkaline and below is acid. Urine is usually acid with a ph of 6.0.

Glucose
This results from a raised blood sugar which leaks into the urine. It occurs in

diabetic clients (glycosuria). Elderly clients need to be screened for this test as they often have few symptoms of diabetes. There is a prevalence in certain racial groups, such as Asian Indians.

Ketones
These can occur as the result of the breakdown of fats to produce energy when the body cannot use sugars, such as diabetes and starvation.

Blood
This can be obvious to the eye or only discovered by testing (haematuria). It can be found with clients on warfarin medication (anti-coagulants), kidney stones, malignancies in the urinary tract, trauma or infection of the urinary tract.

Protein
This can occur after infections, kidney damage, (proteinuria).

Urobilinogen and bilirubin
These are abnormalities associated with liver problems and the client may also have yellow skin (jaundice).

Leucocytes
This is the presence of white cells in the urine and indicate infection.

Nitrates
These are present in the case of infection.

Prostate Gland

The prostate in males is a fleshy organ which is wrapped around the neck of the bladder like a thick collar open at the front. It is made up of glandular tissue and muscle. This organ can enlarge as part of growing older and in very few cases it can be come cancerous.

However, the main problem for males is that it can interfere with the emptying of urine from the bladder, as it can begin to throttle the outlet from the bladder. The collar tightens until it interferes with the flow of urine through the bladder outlet, which can be very painful and distressing for the client.

First signs are when the client starts to experience difficulty in actually passing urine. The flow can be slow and troublesome to get started and may only produce a feeble dribble, it can be worse at night. It also can start with the urge to go to the toilet more and more often and can disturb sleep and activities.

If the bladder is really full it may overflow at night and the client may wet the bed. Sometimes a complete blockage occurs (retention of urine) and they will need emergency treatment involving the insertion of a catheter.

The treatment for an enlarged prostate will depend on the result of the investigations carried out and may be an operation, laser treatment or medication.

Faeces

Faeces are 25% solid matter (undigested food, bacteria, fatty acids) and 75% water, they are normally dark brown, soft and cylindrical in form with an odour from the dead bacteria present in the faeces.

Do you know?

?

Faeces that are passed are formed from the waste products of food in the bowel, which is 1.5 m in length. Special bacteria live in the colon, which can infect the urinary tract if they gain entry through the urethra. At the end of the colon is the rectum where the faeces are stored and these are expelled under voluntary control. The desire to defecate is initiated as a reflex as the entry of food from the stomach causes a movement called peristalsis, along the digestive tract, and by the distension of the colon and rectum. Defecation is normally under voluntary control as the individual can then decide if they want to go (normally in the morning) or leave it to a more convenient time or place with privacy and washing facilities. They are assisted to defecate by anal sphincters (circular muscles) relaxing and the pressure of the abdominal and chest muscles contracting to assist with this expulsion of faeces.

However, the carer may see black tarry stools, pale and fatty looking stools, loose (diarrhoea) stools, undigested food or objects in the faeces, blood and mucus outside the stools. Always observe, save and report any suspicious faeces. The person in charge will check, as it may be due to the medication, illness, chronic disease or a food poisoning infection. The carer may be asked to collect a specimen in a sterile pot from the client. The client may commence a stool or fluid balance chart to record input, output and frequency of stools passed.

Recording

If using a stool chart or care plan, the carer needs to record

- The time
- Amount
- Consistency and any problems
- Their signature and date must also be seen in the care plan

Some clients may need to be asked every day about their bowel movement. There can be problem with confused clients or clients with certain diseases, in getting an accurate history of pain or discomfort. The rectum may need to be examined to ensure it is not blocked with faeces.

Sociocultural factors

Activity 9.7 ■■■■■■■■■■■■■■■■■■■■■■■■■■■

 Consider the many different words that are used for urine and faeces and the different hygienic practices after elimination in the different cultural and social groups.

If your client group consists of many religious and cultural groups, collect information about elimination and their related hygiene practices so you can assist the client before and after elimination.

■■■■■■■■■■■■■■■■■■■■■■■■■■■■■■■■■■■

Some cultural groups may only use their left hand for cleaning their genitals after eliminating and they will keep their right hand for eating. Some older persons may want only staff of the same sex as them to assist them with elimination, and will become very distressed if this is not respected. Some clients may wish to have a jug of water to pour over their genitals after elimination.

Faecal elimination

On admission information from either the client, relatives or carers needs to be collected as regards elimination, the normal pattern and any medication or laxatives taken to prevent diarrhoea or constipation. For most people, defecation is performed at a set time of the day when time and privacy are available.

Constipation

Constipation to some elderly clients may mean they have not been once a day, to others it may be a hard or difficult stool to pass. The clients' diet and intake of food must be noted as well as their religion and cultural group, as it can affect diet choice and hygiene needs. Education on diets and increased fluid intake, as well as encouraging mobility may need to be started after admission.

Do you know?

 The pattern of elimination can vary from three times a day to once every three days. In the young healthy adult the time from when the food is ingested to its output can be three days. In the older person this time can be two weeks. This is due to the sluggish muscular action of the lower digestive tract of the elderly client and may be contributed also by poor diet and lack of mobility.

Consider then the client who is in bed for a long time, or does not have much mobility. It will be more difficult for them to use the abdominal and chest muscles as these have become weaker. They need to be encouraged with passive and active exercises which they will have been shown by the physiotherapists.

Activity 9.8 ■■■■■■■■■■■■■■■■■■■■■■■■■■■■■

 When assisting with care of the client, what would make you think the client could be constipated?

■■■■■■■■■■■■■■■■■■■■■■■■■■■■■■■■■■■■

They may complain or you may observe the following:

- Loss of appetite
- Furred tongue, unpleasant breath
- Abdominal discomfort, straining to pass their stool
- If confused or they have difficulty with speech they will not be able to explain they are constipated and may appear more agitated
- You may notice hard pellet shaped faeces, frequent diarrhoea or watery liquid being passed when they go to the toilet, this may be due to fluid leaking from around impacted faeces.

Activity 9.9 ■■■■■■■■■■■■■■■■■■■■■■■■■■■■

 Can you list the possible causes of constipation?

■■■■■■■■■■■■■■■■■■■■■■■■■■■■■■■■■■■

Your list may include a variety of causes:

- Simple constipation can be caused by low-residue diet or a lack of fluids.
- The toilet may be a long way from the client's room or bed. The toilets may be unsatisfactory due to being dirty, cold and having no toilet paper.
- There may be a lack of privacy when clients come into hospital either caused by lack of curtains or close proximity to other clients in bed. When they are assisted to the toilet, the door may be left open
- Other causes can be due to different medications, immobility from strokes, poor nursing management, bowel obstruction, haemorrhoids with accompanying pain.

Piles (Haemorrhoids)

After bowel movements the carer may be assisting the client with hygiene and notice grape-like projections from their anus, these piles (haemorrhoids) are enlarged varicose veins of the anal canal. They can be seen after the client has strained to pass faeces. The carer needs to report this to the person in charge as the client may need some medication or treatment.

Diarrhoea

This is a change from the pattern of normal stools to more frequent, loose watery bowel movements. It can also be accompanied by abdominal pain and discomfort and disappear in a few days. Sometimes it can last for weeks as the result of a more serious condition.

The causes may be stressful events, such as the move into hospital or a new nursing home. Accidents such as a hip fracture, viral or bacterial infection of the gut can also be the cause of diarrhoea. Some medications such as antibiotics destroy protective bowel bacteria and allow other organisms to cause infection, intolerance of foods and milk feeds. Severe constipation in which watery diarrhoea leaks around the blocked faeces, can cause the onset of diarrhoea or it may be the symptom of a more serious illness.

Activity 9.10 ■■■■■■■■■■■■■■■■■■■■■■■■■■■■

 Consider an older person who may have a chronic or acute illness, who starts having diarrhoea with loss of body fluid. What could happen?

■■■■■■■■■■■■■■■■■■■■■■■■■■■■■■■■■

They can become very dehydrated with the loss of fluid and salts. The insufficient absorption of nutrients from food and can lead to a loss of weight and strength.

The client will need to be encouraged to drink plenty of fluids (oral rehydration programme) and in some serious cases they may need to be started on intravenous therapy to replace fluid lost.

The organisms that can cause intestinal infections (food poisoning) are often from the salmonella family of micro-organism.

The client may have frequent diarrhoea with the need for efficient cleaning of the perineal area and in some cases, cream may need to be applied as the skin can become sore from the faecal matter on the skin.

These infections can spread to other patients from dirty commodes, staff not washing their hands after handling infected linen or faeces, staff not wearing protective equipment (gloves and apron) or not washing their hands before assisting with meals (Fig. 9.6). Therefore every precaution must be taken to prevent cross infection.

Infected clients with diarrhoea

These clients may need to be nursed in isolation (barrier nursed).

Check the organizational policies for dealing with suspected food poisoning outbreaks and barrier nursing. The health care worker will need

Fig. 9.6 Protective clothing when dealing with bodily waste.

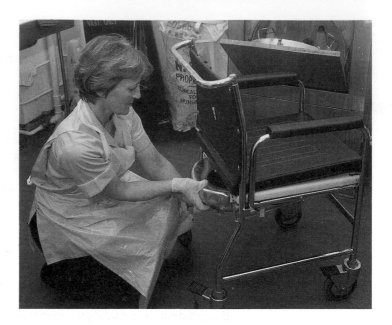

to know what protective equipment to wear (gloves, gown, aprons), correct handwashing procedures, how to dispose of urine or faeces and infected linen, crockery and cutlery and food, and how to clean the room and bed.

A faecal sample

A sample of faeces may be collected by putting a small portion of the faeces into a sterile container and sending to the laboratory for testing.

Stools may also be collected for several days in a container kept in the sluice. Remember to avoid contamination from these faeces. Wear gloves and wash hands afterwards, make sure there is no faecal matter on the outside of the container. An investigation form must be completed and left with the labelled specimen for collection.

Ostomies

Some elderly male and female clients may need surgical intervention for diseases of the bowel or bladder.

With bladder carcinomas, the bladder may need to be removed and the ureters are attached to the bowel and urine is excreted through a uretero-iliostomy into a disposable collection bag on the abdomen.

The bowel may need to be operated on either due to trauma or with a carcinoma and the faeces are then passed directly through an ileostomy or colostomy into a disposable collection bag. This may be a temporary or permanent opening (stoma).

Both operations will need a lot of support for the client and relatives. Scrupulous hygiene must be observed to prevent soreness and irritation around the stoma, or infections when the bags are being changed.

Incontinence

Clients may experience urinary and/or faecal incontinence, however urinary incontinence is the more common

Stokes (1987) defined incontinence as a failure of the mechanisms associated with normal storage and voiding of urine so that involuntary passing of urine occurs in inappropriate places or at an inappropriate time.

Norton & Fader (1994) stated that various studies have shown that between 32 and 55% of people in long-stay hospitals, residential or nursing home care are incontinent of urine or are catheterized.

This obviously causes distress to the client and their relatives and increases the risk of urinary infections. Norton & Fader (1994) stress that the majority of incontinent people can be improved or cured by appropriate selected treatment if this is individually selected for the client.

The control of bladder and bowel continence requires competent urethral and anal sphincter muscles and the ability to inhibit bladder muscle and rectal contraction consciously by the brain. Any of these can be affected by disease or ageing. With increasing age the individual gets less warning and can experience increased urgency of micturition or defecation. Nocturia (rising at night to pass urine) affects some elderly people.

The different types of urinary incontinence are:

- *Stress incontinence*: leakage of urine when coughing, sneezing, laughing or exercising
- *Urge incontinence*: a sudden urgent need to pass urine but not being able to reach the toilet in time
- *Overflow incontinence*: the bladder does not empty completely and the urine then builds up and then overflows from the bladder as a frequent dribbling leakage.

Urinary incontinence

This can be caused by some of the following reasons:

- It may be bladder or urethral problems such as pelvic floor damage from obesity or childbirth
- Urethritis
- Blockage from enlarged prostate or uterine fibroids.
- Incontinence can also be linked to chronic or acute urinary infections leading to urgent or frequent desires to pass urine
- Faecal impaction

■   Mental functions disturbed such as damage to the brain or spinal cord, strokes and Parkinson's Disease.

A plan of care needs to be written after a full and individual assessment of the urinary or faecal incontinence. The condition may be permanent or temporary.

Faecal incontinence

This can be caused by some of the following reasons:

■   Faecal incontinence can be caused by rectal loading with overflow from severe constipation.
■   Other causes can be weak pelvic floor muscles from childbirth or chronic straining over the years, or nerve diseases.
■   Some older persons with dementia may have faecal incontinence due to a physical inability to stop defecation, or because the awareness that this behaviour is inappropriate has been lost.

Overall care

■   Surgery on the pelvic floor or prostate.
■   Pelvic floor exercises, start toileting programmes or bladder training.
■   The multi-disciplinary team have also to consider that toilet difficulties may be due to the elderly client having difficulty using the toilet.
■   Enemas or suppositories may be given to clear the blockage of faeces.

The causes can be that clients are slower at walking or getting out of the chair and they do not reach the toilet in time. Their hands are also less nimble in removing their outer clothing. The use of improved clothing and dressing aids can be worn so they can be removed more easily. The toilet seat may too low, the toilet floor may be dirty and slippery, or the toilet may be up some stairs. Consider obstacles en route, chairs, low tables, inadequate lighting. Also the clients' eyesight may have deteriorated and they may find it difficult to find the toilet, particularly at night. It is important to stress that many older persons may become disorientated at night if they are taking night sedation and will need assistance. Signs should be placed in a prominent position and be large enough to compensate for poor eyesight. These can be symbols or pictorial signs with directional arrows. To assist with these difficulties and to assist with controlling continence, grab rails and raised toilet seats should be available (Fig. 9.7). A commode should be placed by the bed, particularly at night or a urinal for the night. Improved clothing and dressing aids should also be given to clients so they can remove clothing more easily. Carers should help with wheelchairs or give walking aids to clients (refer to Chapter 7) to make continence more easily controllable.

Fig. 9.7 Adapted toilet for client in their own home.

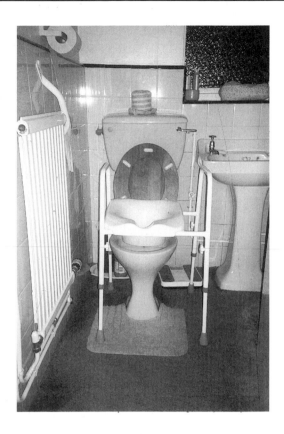

Clients can be embarrassed if not segregated or too few toilets are available. Others stressful situations for clients with continence difficulties include narrow toilets, which do not accommodate walking aids, long corridors, heavy doors with uniform colours that give no clues and bedrooms that are not distinguishable.

Reduce anxiety about continence. 'Mr Smith it is 11.30 in the morning, do you wish to use the toilet before lunch?' By being friendly patient and understanding it will help to reduce anxiety. At night talk quietly and give a reassuring smile.

This loss of control can cause shame in case they soil themselves, denial of their problem is out of fear and embarrassment. Give praise, but do not treat the older person as a child, consider their self respect and dignity. Fear may prompt the client to conceal the situation. Because they have lost control of going to the toilet, they become embarrassed and feel guilty and shameful, and they may attempt to hide soiled underwear. Consider the wearing of old clothes so as not to spoil their good ones. However this can result in a loss of self-esteem and pride in their appearance.

Be patient and tactful, deterioration is not inevitable. There is a need to share disappointments about care. Regular meetings can be a help, when progress can be discussed and 'anger' shared about coping with incontinence all day long.

The carer in the community should be on the lookout for any signs of depression or apathy as this can result in lack of motivation to maintain continence.

Catheters

A catheter is a hollow tube which drains urine from the bladder into a bag. Intermittent catherization either by the nursing staff or the client once a day or two to three times a day may help. Alternatively, the person may have continuous catheterization with a catheter kept in permanently or as a temporary measure. This is called a closed system as the catheter is attached to a drainage tube and bag to collect the urine. However, this should not be the first option if a client is incontinent, due to the high risk of urinary tract infection. These catheters will need to be changed on a regular basis, usually by a nurse. It is important to report if no urine drains from the catheter for a few hours or there is any leakage around the catheter. Always wash hands before and after changing the catheter bag or touching the catheter, and wear gloves.

Catheter care

The genital area should be cleaned regularly with soap and water and any redness, soreness or discharge around the catheter must be reported. Take care when mobilizing clients to avoid pulling on the catheter and ensure it is supported by a stand or a leg attachment (refer to Chapter 7 in *Knowledge to Care* (1994)).

Treatment of incontinence

Individualized toileting programmes

Other options to assist with incontinence, can be individualized toileting programmes using charts to assess the client's individuals pattern of micturition in order to plan toilet regimes and regular toileting regimes at set times. The client must be able to understand and be able to co-operate for some programmes. With many confused patients, timed regular toileting (2–3 hourly) may assist them to keep continent, but this can decrease their independence.

Bladder retraining

Bladder retraining is used if the client has urgency and frequency above seven times a day. This should only be started following the recommendations of a nurse or doctor following a full assessment. The client is asked to hold on and try not to go to the toilet for as long as they can. Medications can be of help with this plan of care. The client should be encouraged to reduce passing urine to about five or six times a day.

It is important to support the client with positive encouragement and help them to maintain their dignity when they start a bladder training programme. This will help them to regain bladder control of urgency and frequency of micturition.

If the client is undergoing a bladder retraining programme, it is important that a record is made of all visits to the toilet or the use of a commode, with the amount of urine passed, plus any times the client is incontinent. The carer has to record the times they assisted patients with regular or individualized toileting programmes in the care plan, or advise the person in charge.

Pelvic floor exercises

These exercises are taught by doctors, physiotherapists and specially trained nurses (continence nurse specialists) to help strengthen the muscles and to help the client hold urine. The pelvic floor muscles stretch like a hammock from the pubic bone in front to the bottom of the spine. They hold the bladder, womb and bowel in place and help to close the bladder outlet and back passage. The muscles of the pelvic floor are normally kept firm and slightly tense to stop leaks of urine from the bladder or faeces from the bowel (Fig. 9.8).

When the client passes urine or has a bowel movement, the pelvic floor muscles relax and afterwards they tighten again to restore control. These muscles can become weak and sag because of childbirth, lack of exercise, and as one of the stages of getting older. The weakening of the muscles can lead to less control and the client may leak urine after exercise, if they cough, sneeze or laugh (stress incontinence).

Depending on the level of weakness, clients can see good results. But it can take several months for this to occur. Clients need support and encouragement at all times. Clients can often see good results in many cases after a few weeks, if they follow the exercises every day.

Continence aids

Sometimes, it is not possible to regain continence completely, but with planning and good products the client and can have an improved life-style which can assist them to lead more independent lives at home with their relatives. However, no product is perfect for everybody, so assessment is needed by a continence nurse specialist. People are different sizes, shapes, have different elimination patterns and personal preferences. The aids are chosen depending on the degree of incontinence, mobility, dexterity and size of the client.

The family and health care assistants may need to be involved with the assessment as some aids are disposable, some washable, some for the bed, some for the body. Advice can be sought from the continence nurse spe-

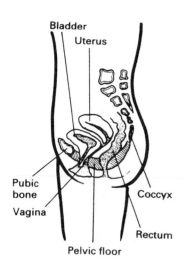

Bladder

Uterus

Pubic bone

Vagina

Coccyx

Rectum

Pelvic floor

Fig. 9.8 Side-view of female pelvic floor muscles (courtesy of Lurex Synthelabo).

cialist in each area about a toileting programme (exercises or bladder training) and about these aids.

Incontinence aids may consist of pants with a pouch (e.g. Kanga) stretch pants, pads with waterproof backing held in place with lightweight stretch knickers for male or females, or all-in-one diapers worn by clients in bed, in particular for night-time use. If the client is going home and there is still a continence problem, to assist the carer, a bed protection either as disposable or washable pads needs to be considered. Incontinence pads and draw sheets over plastic sheets, or washable pads (Kylie sheets) are often used.

Before discharge from hospital, disposal of these aids and cleaning material for urine and faecal contamination needs to be discussed, in addition to a laundering service for bed linen for clients at home. Other suggestions that the continence nurse specialist can put forward include hand-held urinals for clients in wheelchairs and disposable male urinals (Reddy bottle, Simcare) or commodes for the bedroom (refer to chapter 7, Supported Living).

Should the client be confined to a chair or a bed, they are also assessed as being at risk from pressure sores using a scale, for example the Waterlow or Norton scale. Specialist mattresses or cushions can also be used (refer to Chapter 10, Hygiene, Comfort and Rest).

Support and encouragement

The importance of supporting the client and carer with these aids, showing discretion and tact, and also maintaining the privacy of the client at all times is crucial. The client may feel very ashamed and distressed, since they feel they have lost their dignity and independence by using these aids.

These aids can also affect their sexual and personal relationships. They may worry if they smell or fear the risk of accidents. Clients who wear catheters need to be reassured that they do not need to stop their previous sexual relationships and they should be encouraged to continue after discharge by being provided with accurate information by a qualified nurse. For females, the use of bidets or adaptations for the toilet to wash and dry the perineal area frequently may help to reassure the client.

Hygiene

Personal cleanliness with incontinent clients is very important. Disposable wipes with special skin cleanser or ordinary mild soap and water, with careful drying and a simple barrier cream may be used. Depending on the organizational procedure, it is important to report any soreness, redness, or broken skin, or if a pressure sore is developing when assisting with post-elimination hygiene (refer to Chapter 10, Hygiene). Urine is mildly irritant to the skin and with the moisture from wet linen or clothing and friction if the client is roughly dragged along the bed, abrasions of the skin can occur.

To avoid smells, it is important to change wet clothing, pads or wet bed linen as soon as possible. Urine or faecal spillage must be cleaned up immediately and soiled pads and disposable cleaning materials should be put in airtight bins or a sealed bag as soon as possible. Consider sprays or air fresheners in the room or by the bed after caring for the client if there is a smell, as it will be distressing and embarrassing in many cases for clients and their relatives.

Activity 9.11 ■■■■■■■■■■■■■■■■■■■■■■■■■■

 Who do you think are the other members of the team that can assist with elimination needs?

■■■■■■■■■■■■■■■■■■■■■■■■■■■■■■■■■■

Continence nurse specialists
These have specialist knowledge of helping people with incontinence problems.

Health visitor/district nurse
Health visitors have specialist training with elderly clients and district nurses are involved with the management of continence in the community.

Dietitian
A dietitian can advise on diet and help with diarrhoea and constipation, diabetic diets, low salt diets, reducing diets and undernourished patients (refer to Chapter 8, Nutrition).

Occupational therapists
These assist with toilet aids, dressing aids, mobility aids and also help with socializing activities.

Physiotherapists
These help with mobility, passive and active exercises, pelvic floor muscle assessment and exercises.

Dentists
These can examine and treat the mouth or provide new dentures to assist with improved eating and drinking.

Chiropodists (podiatrists)
These examine and treat foot problems to assist with improved mobility.

Optician/hearing aids technician
These examine and provide improved aids to assist with communication.

Social workers
They advise on financial help and organize modifications to the home, such as downstairs toilets and a laundry service with the local authority.

Psychologist/community psychiatric nurse (CPN)
These people can help the client who has learning disabilities or who is confused about toilet training.

Further help

Some clients may be assessed at a day hospital and their ongoing management may be as a day patient. This may mean they do not have to be admitted into a nursing home for long term care as their continence may be treatable.

The multi-disiplinary team will also consist of the medical team. These include GPs, hospital specialists such as a urologist, gynaecologists, geriatrician or gastroenterologists, to assist with assessment, planning, implementation and evaluation for the individual client's elimination needs.

Health and safety

Consider yourself and the client.

Are you trained in patient handling to mobilize clients or assist them safely on the commode, or bedpan? You should be trained and regularly reviewed in order to protect your back and to prevent harm and discomfort to the clients.

Are you up to date with your immunizations? Check with your GP or your occupational health department since you are handling body fluids.

Do you know the infection control procedures for urine and faeces; particularly concerning protective equipment and if there is any spillage? Do you know you always need to check the care plan before assisting clients with elimination, as they may need hoists or two staff to mobilize them?

When walking clients you always need to ensure the passageway is clear of obstacles and is well lit. Take your time, and always check their walking aids.

When reaching the toilet, you need to know if they need to have a toilet aid to raise the height, particularly if they have osteoarthritis. Offer clients the hand rails in the wall, as it will also help with mobilization.

You need to know if you need to stay with the client during elimination. What did the care plan say? If you leave the client, show them the call bell, or check frequently. But remember privacy – do not leave the door open.

Would you know what to do if the door was locked and you could not open it? Check the procedures.

Would you know what to do if the client collapsed in the toilet or if the client required assistance with breathing and circulation until help arrived? What is the emergency number of your area and where is the emergency equipment in your area of work? Are you trained in cardiopulmonary resuscitation and are you aware of your organizations procedure?

Do not leave the client on the toilet or commode too long as the circulation to the skin of the buttocks will be affected along with reddening of the skin. It can also lead to the breakdown of the skin and the risk of pressure sores and infection. If you leave the client on the commode, place the commode facing the bed in case they feel faint and fall forward.

Ensure you leave the toilet and floor clean; that the contents of the commode, urinals and bedpans are disposed of correctly and that they are cleaned according to your organizational procedures.

After removing your gloves and aprons, wash your hands again before carrying out any other procedures for clients.

Summary

Elimination is an essential activity of living. For many clients it will require assistance to meet their elimination and post-elimination needs, many of these clients would have been independent with this activity before admission. Losing this independence can lead to a loss of self-esteem and embarrassment. It is important therefore, that the carer maintains privacy and dignity during these activities with the client.

Observation while assisting the client and reporting of any problems is essential for providing ongoing care to meet their individual needs. The client may also be embarrassed to use the commode or bedpan. However, they can be assisted to use a wheelchair or walking aids to the toilet and to dispose of their own body waste.

Remember at all times the clients' and other carers' health and safety needs and always check the care plan before assisting with elimination.

References

DHSS (1981) *Growing Older*. HMSO, London.

Norton, M. & Fader, C. (1994) Incontinence. *Elderly Care*, November/December, **6** (6), 23.

Stokes, G. (1987) *Incontinence and Inappropriate Urinating*. Winslow Press, Bicester.

Voluntary Euthanasia Society (1992) *Your Ultimate Choice*. Souvenir Press, London.

Further reading

Addison, R. (1996) Faecal incontinence. *Nurse Prescriber/Community Nurse*, January, 29.

Brown, C. (1994) Community Centre (Continence Supplement). *Nursing Times*, 26 January, **90** (4), 86.

Caffrey, R. (1994) Stress incontinence, a personal plan. *Nursing Times*, 26 January, **90** (4), 84.

Continence Foundation (1995) *Pelvic Floor Exercises*, Leaflet available from, Continence Foundation, The Basement, 2 Doughty Street, London WC1N 2PH.

Continence Foundation (1994) *Continence Guide, All you need to know.* Available from, The Continence Foundation, 2 Doughty Street, London WC1N 2PH.

Counsel and Care for the Elderly. *A Positive Approach to Incontinence for Older People.* Available free, from Counsel and Care for the Elderly, Twyman House, 16 Bonny Street, London NW1 9PG (SAE).

Fader, M. (1994) From wheelchair to toilet. *Nursing Times*, 13 April, **90** (15), 76.

Fader, M.J., Barnes, K.E., Malone-Lee, J.G. & Cottingden, A.M. (1987) Choosing the right garment. *Nursing Times*, 15 April, **83** (15), 85–87.

Fader, M. & Norton, C. (1995) *Caring for Continence, A Care Assistants guide.* Hawker, London. Available from, Hawker Publications, 13 Park House, 140 Battersea Park Road, London SW11 4NB.

Getcliffe, K. (1995) Long-term catheter use in the community. *Elderly Care*, June **7** (3), 21.

Gould, D. (1994). Catheters, Keeping on tract. *Nursing Times*, 5 October, **90** (40), 58.

Healey, F. (1994) Does flooring type affect risk of injury in older patients? *Nursing Times*, 6 July, **90** (27), 40.

Help the Aged (1995) *Incontinence.* Advice leaflet available from, Help the Aged, St James's Walk, London EC1R 0BE.

Lloyd, C. (1993) Making sense of reagent strip urine test. *Nursing Times*, 1 December, **89** (48), 32.

Narzarko, L. (1993) Preventing constipation. *Elderly Care*, March/April, **5** (2), 32.

Pearson, P. (1994) Pelvic floor exercises, muscle control. *Nursing Times*, 9 March, **90** (10), 64.

Ross, J. (1994) A plan of action. *Nursing Times*, 6 July, **90** (27), 64.

Sandvik, H. (1994) Devising a severity index for incontinence. *Nursing Times*, 11 May, **90** (19), 11.

Simpla Plastics (1995) *You and Your Catheter.* Available free from, Simpla Plastics Ltd, FREEPOST, Cardiff CF4 ZZ.

Turner, T. (1994) Muscle control. *Nursing Times*, 9 March **90** (10), 64.

Wells, M. (1994) Achieving good care. *Nursing Times*, 26 October, **90** (43), 43.

Williams, K. (1995) Developments in continence care. Constipation in old age. *Elderly Care*, October/November, **7** (5), 19.

Wright, S. (1992) *Nursing the Older Patient*, Chapter 12. Chapman & Hall, London.

Useful addresses

Association for Continence Advice
Winchester House
Kennington Park
Cranmer Road
The Oval
London SW9 6EG

Age Concern England
Bernard Sunley House
Pitcairn Road
Mitcham
Surrey CR4 3LL

Continence Foundation
The basement
2 Doughty Street
London WC1N 2PH

Disabled Living Foundation
346 Kensington High Street
London W14 8NS

Health Education Authority
Hamilton House
Mabledon Place
London WC1H 9TX

Help the Aged England
St James Walk
London EC1R 0BE

Help the Aged Scotland
33 Castle Street
Edinburgh EH2 3DN

Help the Aged Wales
1 Park Grove
Cardiff CF1 3B

InconTact,
The Dene Centre
Castle Farm Road
Newcastle-upon-Tyne NE3 1PH

Chapter 10
Hygiene, Comfort and Rest
Christine McMahon

Overview

In this chapter the clients' hygiene needs, including mouth, hair and nail care, will be discussed as well as how to help them to be comfortable and rest effectively. The chapter discusses the following:

■ The importance of individualized care and the care of the clients' clothes.
■ The overall comfort of the client considering the effect of ageing on the skin and the importance of pressure area care and correct positioning of the client, identifying those most at risk.
■ The causes and prevention of pressure sores with the various aids used in their prevention.
■ The causes of pain and how to minimize its effects and the importance of rest for the well-being of the client.

Key words

Hygiene, skin care, ageing, care plan, immobile, preparation of equipment, privacy, choice, self-esteem, oral hygiene, observation of skin, safety, pressure areas, positioning, pain/stress relief, insomnia, sleep pattern.

Skin care and personal hygiene of the older person

As people age, their skin tends to become thinner, to change in texture and become more fragile.
    This is due to various factors:

■ Collagen, the fibrous substance which supports the skin tissue is less elastic and therefore skin looses its elasticity and sags.
■ Dehydration of the skin is more of a problem leading to a tendency towards dry skin. The production of an oily substance called sebum, which is produced in the sebaceous glands under the skin, is reduced. This protective oil prevents water loss from the skin.

As the structure of the skin changes, the rate that skin cells are renewed slows down. All this results in skin that becomes thinner, dry and more likely to breakdown and should it do so, it will take a long time to heal. As skin becomes dry, itching (pruritus) can occur. There is also an increase in the pigmentation (colouring matter in the skin) these are sometimes known as 'age spots' and can often be seen on the back of the hands of the older person. Dark warts may also appear on the trunk of the client. These are quite common in the older person, but should they bleed or become inflamed they must be brought to the attention of the person in charge or the doctor.

The older person needs a well-balanced diet that includes plenty of fluids, protein, vitamins and minerals (refer to Chapter 8, Nutrition). Circulation is important too, as this aids the nutrients and oxygen which all cells need, to be circulated around the body. Skin cells that are deprived of oxygen and nutrients are in danger of dying and developing a pressure sore (necrotic tissue). Careful attention to personal hygiene has many benefits to the client.

Activity 10.1 ■

List the benefits to the client when their hygiene needs are fully met.

■ ■

Your list could include many different aspects of the client' needs as set out below.

Making the client feel better

Just the fact that the client has experienced a pleasant, relaxing bath can improve the client's 'feel good' factor and increase their self-esteem. If the bath contains rehydrating perfumed oils, these all help the client to relax.

Prevention of infection

Keeping the skin clean prevents *cross-infection*, especially by the client having the opportunity to wash their hands after using the toilet or before eating. Careful hygiene will help to prevent *urinary tract infection* in the female client. By meticulous perineal care, (area between urethra/outlet from the bladder and the anus/outlet from the bowel) bacteria will be prevented from travelling up the urethra to the bladder and causing a urinary tract infection (cystitis). The older person is more vulnerable to infection with an incidence of the increased risk of urinary tract infection in females over the age of 65 years. Cleansing should always be undertaken from front to back to prevent contamination of the urethra. Washing in warm soapy water and then careful drying can help to destroy bacteria.

Encourage the client to drink plenty of fluids (two litres per day). This will also help to prevent an infection by regularly flushing the urinary tract.

Careful and regular mouthcare will help to prevent *mouth infections.*

Therapeutic effects

Additions to the bath of a dermatological bath oil prior to going to bed, can have a soothing effect on dry and itchy skin. By adding these oils to the bath it enables all parts of the body to be treated, especially the client's back, if they are self-caring. Soaking in a bath oil for 15–20 minutes can be most beneficial as specialist oils can help to restore lost moisture and flexibility of the skin. However, care must be taken that a client is not encouraged to soak in a bath without a rehydrating oil as the skin will become dehydrated and dry.

Note: If oils are added to the bath water, there is a danger of the client slipping, therefore a non-slip bath mat must be used and the client assisted at all times.

Cultural needs

Hygiene can feature in different cultures and religions and it may be important for a client to wash in particular way or at a specific time. Carers should always be aware of these needs and assist the client when necessary in order for these needs to be fulfilled.

Bathing

The way in which hygiene needs are met will depend on the clients' wishes, their level of mobility and independence. The care plan will indicate whether the client should undertake an assisted wash in the bathroom or in bed, and whether any bathing aid, such as a hoist should be used.

It is important to consider the clients' overall health and mobility. For instance a client with rheumatoid arthritis may have severe limitations of movement in all limbs. A client who has difficulty breathing while lying down will be unable to lie flat during a bed bath and the carer will need to take this into account during the procedure.

Activity 10.2   ■

 List the clients, whose bathing procedure needed adaptations with the reasons why.

■ ■

Negotiation with the client should identify the time for bathing, to suit both the client and carer.

Case study 1

Jane was a client at home, who required help with bathing due to her broken arm. The carer was planned to arrive for 09.00 hrs to assist Jane. But there were times when the carer was delayed and Jane would have prepared all her clothes and toilet articles for 09.00 hrs only to be kept waiting. It proved difficult to meet Jane's needs for an early wash so the carer helped Jane to plan her own care and adapted her room. With the addition of some washing aids Jane was able to wash herself at the time she wished, thereby keeping to her own routine.

Safety

Safety during bathing of the older person is an important consideration as they can be frail and less mobile. Special equipment may be required, such as grab handles, bath boards or seats to assist the client getting in and out of the bath. The occupational therapist can give the appropriate advice to the client and arrange for adaptations to be made (Figs 10.1 and 10.2).

There is a diminished sensation of temperature in the older person and they do not always register the temperature of bath water. Always run cold water in first, then the hot and check the temperature before the client gets in to prevent scalds.

Fig. 10.1 Bathing aids.

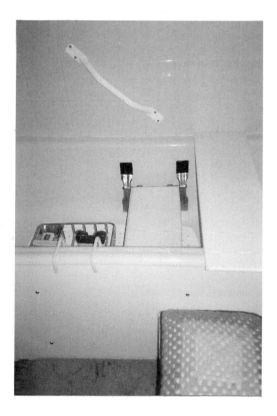

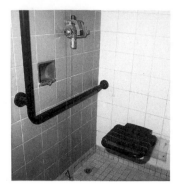

Fig. 10.2 Adapted shower.

If the client is independent enough to leave alone, always ensure they have some means easily to hand to call for assistance should it be required. It is recommended to use a bath mat both in and outside the bath to prevent the client slipping.

Have all the necessary toiletries, clean clothes and linen ready before undressing and washing the client. Preparation is important to prevent care becoming fragmented and disorganized. This can give the impression of not caring for a client and not fully understanding their needs. Apart from leading to unsafe practices it can lead to the client becoming frustrated and upset. Good preparation will not only give the impression of efficiency, but will save time in the long run. Toiletries must not be shared between clients, since to do so would violate clients' rights and could lead to cross-infection.

A different flannel and towel should be used for face and upper part of the body than the perineal area and buttocks to prevent contamination and possible infection.

Water should be changed whenever it becomes too cold or soapy and after washing the client's perineum and buttocks.

It may be local practice for the carer to wear a plastic apron while washing a client, in which case the reason for doing so should be explained to the client.

Washing bowls are a potential source of infection. Each client should have their own bowl, which should be washed and dried after use and stored singly upside down.

Always consider the dignity and privacy of the client and ensure that doors or curtains are closed.

Aim to work with the client when meeting their specific needs. Find out the client's needs, involve them in their own care, empower them by giving choice and control, and ensure the client is not interrupted while washing.

You can refer to other books for detailed descriptions of how to wash a client, for instance, Chapter 8, Hygiene, *Knowledge to Care* (1994).

Oral hygiene

The aim of mouth care is to keep the mouth moist, free from infection and prevent the build up of plaque deposits.

Inadequate mouth care of the older person can contribute to poor eating habits as it affects the appetite and pleasurable experience of enjoying a meal. The senses of taste and smell are decreased, resulting in a reduced response by the body to food. Normally when food is smelt or tasted the flow of saliva increases, this saliva moistens the mouth and also helps to destroy bacteria.

Teeth are important and need care, they enable the client to bite and chew normal food. Without teeth the diet may well have to be modified, therefore restricting the older person's choice of food.

Oral care for the older person is most important, as already stated their resistance to infection is reduced and if oral hygiene needs are not met then mouth infection or bleeding and gum (peridontal) disease can occur. This results in discomfort for the client and the possible loss of teeth and halitosis (bad breath).

Activity 10.3 ■

 Consider the way in which you care for your teeth.

■ ■

Your list may include:

- Cleaning teeth night and morning, after each meal
- Use of dental floss

- Cleaning and soaking dentures or plates
- Visiting the dentist for regular check-ups

When considering the older person, any remaining teeth should be brushed night and morning with a soft toothbrush and toothpaste. The handle of a toothbrush can be built up to make it easier to grip for the client who has difficulty in gripping a toothbrush, for example those with severe arthritis.

Dentures should be removed daily and carefully cleaned to remove any food deposits. The gums and tongue can be gently brushed with a soft toothbrush dipped in mouthwash to freshen the mouth and to remove any coating from the tongue and gums. Care should be taken to clean the area between the gum and cheek to remove any deposits of food. If any soreness is detected, inform the person in charge, as this can lead to infection and difficulty in eating, with a loss of appetite.

Regular dental check-ups by the dentist are advised. This helps in the early detection of problems or disease, such as mouth cancer, which occurs more frequently in the older person (Fairclough, 1993).

Activity 10.4 ■

 List the different ways that you have met clients' oral hygiene needs.

■ ■

Hand and foot care

Finger nails should be cut or filed according to the client's wishes. A female client may require assistance to varnish her nails. It is important to try and maintain the client's own routine as much as possible. The client's own nail brush may be used to clean dirty nails.

Toe nails are easier to cut using nail clippers as they tend to be thicker and stronger than finger nails and should follow the shape of the toe.

Special care should be taken when cutting toe nails to avoid damaging the surrounding skin. In some organizations this can only be undertaken by a registered nurse or podiatrist. Always consult the person in charge or the podiatrist before attempting to cut toe nails. Clients with poor circulation or diabetes are at particular risk, as any break in the skin could become infected and take a long time to heal.

Do you know?

During an average person's life time, feet walk approximately four times around the world.

Women tend to suffer from more foot problems than men due to wearing high heels.

Prior to cutting toe nails, soak the feet in a bowl of warm water containing a rehydrating bath oil. This will help to soften the nails and also help to remove any dry, hard callused skin when gently rubbed with a well soaped pumice stone. After nails are cut, rinse and dry feet, taking special care between the toes and then apply an emollient cream.

Foot care is important as some older people find it difficult to reach their feet, so they require the help of a carer. In addition to meeting the physical needs of the client, foot care involves time spent with the client which has a psychological benefit. Not only will it increase their overall comfort and sense of well-being, it will also give the client the feeling of being cared for and the opportunity to talk to the carer (Fig. 10.3).

Hair care

Try to maintain the client's normal routine. For example, visit the hairdresser once a month for a trim or perm. Many hairdressers will visit the clients in their own home or a residential setting. Always ensure the identity and qualifications of a hairdresser before entry to a client's home (Fig. 10.4).

Self-esteem is a most important consideration. We all know how we feel should our hair be unkempt or dirty. Some clients may find it difficult to brush and care for their own hair, so will require assistance. If the client is unable to express an opinion the relatives should be consulted (refer to Chapter 8, in *Knowledge to Care* (1994) for further details concerning washing and general care of the hair).

Make-up and cosmetics

One of the aims of care is to maintain the client's normal routine and control over their own care. Many female clients may wish to express their individuality and sexuality by wearing make-up or jewellery. Always

Fig. 10.3 Client
receiving foot care at
home.

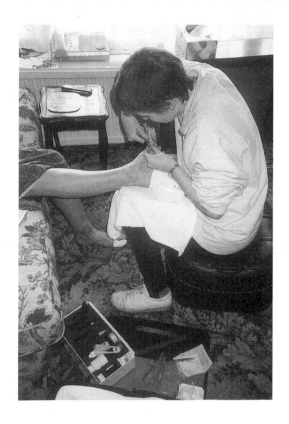

Fig. 10.4 Client having
hair washed and set at
home.

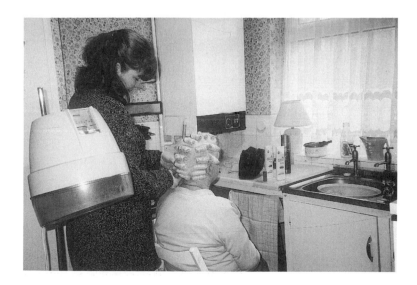

consider the finer details of this aspect of care. Does your client want moisturising cream on their face, wear eye shadow or lipstick?

Each client will have her own preferences and this may involve others in keeping them supplied with their particular requirements. The use of make-up and jewellery helps a client to express their sexuality and the way in which they are perceived by others. Some female clients may need assistance to remove facial hair, this procedure needs discretion and consideration, as it can be a source of embarrassment for the client.

Shaving

Male clients usually shave their face daily and may need assistance to undertake this task. Morale and self-esteem can be improved by shaving, and to some male clients it may be very important that they shave once a day. For some clients their preferences may be influenced by religious or cultural needs and these must always be respected.

It is best to use the type of razor that the client is used to, however it is important that electric razors are not shared as they can be a source of cross-infection; especially blood-borne infections. If the client wishes to have a wet shave, then a safety razor must be used, taking care to dispose of any blades or disposable razors safely in a sharps box.

Dressing and supply of personal clothes and linen

When helping an older person to dress who, for example, does not have the full use of both arms, or someone who has suffered a stroke, always remove clothing from the unaffected side first. Then when replacing clothes, put the affected arm in first, this will make it easier. Always remove clothes carefully over a client's head taking off their spectacles first should they be wearing them.

The occupational therapist can help with advice concerning dressing aids and adaptations that can be made to clothes (Fig. 10.5). These aids will enable the client to dress and undress themselves and maintain a degree of independence and control over their own care (refer to Chapter 7, Supported Living).

Clients should have the opportunity to choose which colours and clothes they wish to wear. This gives the client the chance to express their own mood and feelings of the day. The choice of colours can have a beneficial effect on the way we feel. It has been found that wearing the colour green can have a calming and reassuring effect on the person.

Activity 10.5 ■

 Describe your favourite outfit, and give the reason why it makes you 'feel good'.

■ ■

Fig. 10.5 Dressing aids.

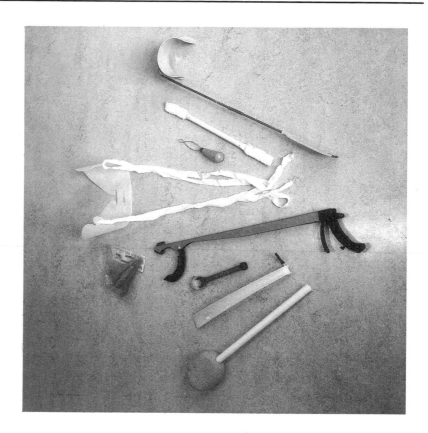

Clothes can reflect our culture, life-style, religion, status, belonging to a club or association and our overall sense of well-being and mood. The type of clothes can influence how others treat a client and affect mood, confidence or motivation (Goodwin, 1995). Always try and maintain a selection of clothes so that there is a degree of choice for the client each day. Cupboards and drawers should be accessible to the client to ensure their independence when selecting their clothes. A suitably placed mirror can help to promote a better dress sense for the client.

Check clothes for general maintenance, for example is there a button missing or has the hem come undone? Consider the correct care of clothing, should it be dry cleaned or washed, and if so how? Clothes are an expensive commodity and we must enable the client to care for them in accordance to the manufacturers instructions. It can help if each client has their own labelled laundry bag for soiled clothes. Some organizations have a designated person who has the overall responsibility for the care and laundry of personalized clothing (Goodwin, 1995).

In the institutional or residential setting it is advisable that clients' clothing is discreetly named in order for the correct clothes to be given to the correct client. Perhaps relatives can help with this and any new clothing is given to the client already labelled.

Case study 2

Pete was up and about and had been in hospital for a week. He was most unco-operative when asked if he would take a bath and although he had not had a bath for some time, he refused.

Later in the day while one of the carers was talking to Pete, he said that he would like a bath but, because he did not have any clean clothes to put on afterwards he felt it inappropriate to have one. The carer then made enquiries as to how clean clothes could be obtained. When clean clothes were given to Pete, he was more than willing to have a bath and his hair washed. Following the bath and donning clean clothes Pete was a different person, he was more confident and entered into conversations willingly and it was obvious that his self-esteem was restored.

Footwear

Do not forget to check the client's footwear is in good repair and safe. Shoes that need repairing or have a very slippery sole can be a danger to the older person who is unsteady on their feet. Shoes should also be the correct size, comfortable and give support. It may well be of benefit for the client to wear shoes during the day – then change into slippers for the evening. The occupational therapist may be able to help in obtaining shoes with easy fasteners for the client with poor manual dexterity. There are shoe companies which specialize in supplying foot wear for swollen and arthritic feet. Facilities should be available for the client to clean their own shoes or have this done for them. In a residential setting there may be a resident who can undertake this for others less able, and get a sense of worth and satisfaction in doing so.

Bed linen

The care of bed linen may need special attention if it has been soiled with faeces, urine or blood. The carer should wear gloves to dispose of the excess faeces down the toilet, before placing the linen in a designated polythene bag in accordance with your operational policy. Usually this is a red dissolvable plastic bag that can be put directly into a washing machine. A domestic washing machine can be used and the linen washed separately from other bed linen or clothing at a high temperature. Incontinent clients at home who do not have a washing machine, may be entitled to a local authority bed linen collection and washing facility.

Pressure area care

There has been much written about pressure sores including the causes, prevention and treatment and it is impossible to cover all these issues within the scope of this chapter. Therefore, the reader is recommended to cheek the further reading at the end of the chapter.

Prevention is better than cure

Pressure sores are expensive in all aspects; discomfort, pain and suffering for the client. The additional costs of treatment and a possible prolonged stay in hospital can also deprive the client of their home and family. In extreme cases, pressure sores can cause death, as they become infected and septicaemia can occur.

Do you know?

The average person makes 400 spontaneous movements of some kind during an eight hour night. Elderly clients who made 225 did not develop pressure sores (Blicharz, 1979).

If we feel uncomfortable due to being in one position, this message is transferred to our brain and we then change position. However if the client is unable to feel or comprehend the discomfort, due to nerve or brain damage, or they cannot change position due to frailty or despondency, the prolonged pressure can cause a pressure sore.

Pressure sores occur when an area of tissue has been deprived of oxygen and nutrients. Immobility is a major factor and it is known that the risk is increased in the older person over 65 years of age.

Activity 10.6 ■

Pull your sleeve up and place your arm on a firm surface, lean your other elbow on it and press down.
How does it feel? Yes, it is uncomfortable, but keep on pressing for a couple of minutes.
Now remove your elbow – what do you see?

■ ■

On first removing your elbow you will have a cool, paler area, which will then quickly redden. Your elbow as the hard object has put pressure on your skin and compressed it against the underlying bone. This results in the small tubes carrying blood (capillaries) being squashed and preventing the flow of blood, making the area paler. When the pressure is removed the body quickly realizes that an area has been deprived of blood, and to compensate, the blood vessels enlarge to allow an increased flow of blood to the area (hyperaemic reaction). If you place the back of a bent finger above the reddened area it will feel hot, due to the increased blood flow. If your skin is dark then it may be difficult to distinguish a reddened area but, you will still feel the heat from it.

Do not rub the affected area, as this will only interrupt the body's response to the prolonged pressure and reduced blood supply. It has been shown that rubbing can damage the small blood capillaries and cause a pressure sore.

Observe your arm in 15 minutes time and there should not be any trace of the reddened area.

When changing the position of a client, always observe pressure areas for signs of redness or heat, any area that remains affected for longer than 45 minutes is in danger of developing tissue damage and a pressure sore. Any signs of redness or heat must be reported to the person in charge.

Activity 10.7 ■

Can you list the areas most at risk where pressure sores may occur?

■ ■

Your list may include;

- Buttocks (sacral area)
- Heels
- Hip (ischial tuberosity, pelvis)
- Ankle

Fig. 10.6 Areas prone to pressure.

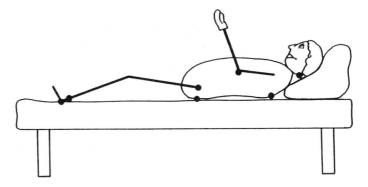

Other areas include head, spine, shoulder, sides of the knees (Fig. 10.6).

These bony prominences of an immobile client are where *prolonged pressure* restricts the blood flow to the tissues, preventing oxygen and nutriments feeding the cells (ischaemia) and the removal of waste products from the tissues. This ischaemic area will result in the breakdown of tissue (necrosis) and the formation of an ulcer/pressure sore (decubitis ulcer).

Shearing occurs when the client who is sitting up slips down the bed. The skin stays where it is, but the underlying bone and tissue moves down with the weight of the client. This causes the capillaries to be stretched inhibiting the flow of blood to the skin.

Activity 10.8 ■

Place your lower arm on the table with your elbow at the edge. Press down hard on your arm and pull it towards you and over the end of the table. You can see that your skin has stayed in the same place, while your bones (radius and ulna) have moved.

■ ■

The most common places for shearing to occur are the buttocks and heels.

Activity 10.9   ■

Can you list the clients most at risk of developing a pressure sore?

■ ■

Your list could include clients that are:

- Immobile
- Incontinent
- Too thin or fat
- Oedematous (excess fluid in the tissues)
- Confused or heavily sedated
- Unconscious

- Paralysed, stroke victims with a loss of pain sensation and movement
- Diabetics
- Suffering from poor circulation or nutrition
- Depressed

Oedema is the presence of excess fluid in the tissues which gravitates down to the lowest part of the body, i.e. ankles in the client who is up and about and sits in chair. While the client who is confined to bed, oedema gravitates down to the sacral area. Oedema increases the risk of pressure sores, as it interferes with the transportation of oxygen and nutriments needed by the skin tissue.

Incontinence also increases the risk of the development of a pressure sore. The damp sheets increase friction on the skin and urine weakens the skin, which in turn increases the risk of infection and the development of a pressure sore (refer to Chapter 9). There are various assessment tools and scales to assess the overall physical and mental levels of a client resulting in a score to give the risk factor of a client developing a pressure sore. For example the Waterlow or Norton scales.

Activity 10.10   ■

Describe any assessment tool used in your work area.

■ ■

A risk assessment tool could include the general state of health relating to levels of:

- Mobility
- Activity
- Nutrition
- Anaemia

- Fluid intake
- Consciousness
- Incontinence
- Depression

Principles of pressure area care

Relieve pressure
Frequent changes of the client's position need to take place about every two hours if they are using a standard mattress. In the case of the client

confined to a chair, encourage sit ups at frequent intervals, for example half hourly. Remember that pressure sores can occur in *all* immobile clients, that includes not only those confined to bed, but also those who are immobile and sitting in chairs for any length of time.

A turning chart is helpful in planning and recording the positions, for instance you can plan for the client to be sitting up at meal times. Client handling needs to be careful to prevent any drag on buttocks or heels as the client is assisted up the bed to prevent friction (refer to Chapter 11, Mobility).

Bed linen must be kept clean and dry, and care taken when making a bed to keep sheets tight and wrinkle free. When making beds, always remember to leave the top bed clothes loose to enable the client to move and change position easily without restriction. Some clients prefer duvets as they find them lighter and allow easier movement.

Skin hygiene needs to be careful and thorough especially in the case of the incontinent client, or one who is perspiring profusely

An adequate intake of protein, vitamins, zinc, iron and fluids is required to maintain a *nutritious diet* (refer to Chapter 8, Nutrition).

Pressure relieving aids, can benefit the client, these include specialized mattresses, beds and cushions.

Activity 10.11 ■

 Describe the pressure relieving aids that are in use in your care environment.

■ ■

If possible, always include the client when planning care, so that they understand something about the prevention of pressure sores and can have a certain amount of control in preventing them.

Minimizing clients' discomfort and pain

One of the most common questions asked of many clients is: '*Are you feeling comfortable?*'

But the words comfortable and comfort can have many meanings, and have different meanings to different people.

Activity 10.12 ■

 Write down what the word comfort means to you.

■ ■

Your list may include:

■ Putting someone into a 'good' position
■ Free from pain

- Relief from anxiety
- Feeling 'at one' with the world
- Stress or trouble free.

According to the *Oxford Concise Dictionary* comfort means relief of affliction, physical well-being, being comfortable, soothe in grief, consolation, console.

From these definitions you can see that comfort has an impact on the *physical*, *psychological* and *biological* aspects of the client. For example:

- Putting someone in a good/suitable position could meet a *physical need*
- Relief of affliction would meet a *biological need*
- Consolation would meet a *psychological need*

You are well aware that it is difficult to divide needs into these three categories, as many times they will overlap. There must have been numerous occasions that you have put someone into a more comfortable position, thus meeting a physical need, and at the same time meeting a biological need by reducing discomfort. You will also meet their psychological need by making them 'feel' better, and encouraging them to think of something else and above all, spending time with them.

Maslow, a psychologist in the 1970s categorized a person's needs into a hierarchy. Physiological needs are at the base, then safety and security, love and belonging, self-esteem and finally self-actualization.

self-actualization
self-esteem
love and belonging
safety and security
physiological needs

Each lower layer of need must be met before meeting others.

Imagine you are in pain, what would your first priority be? It would be to remove the pain first, and not to put on clean night wear for your visitors, thinking about your self-esteem.

The consideration of these needs is included in the vocational qualification O Unit and promoting equality for the client and should be reflected in all the care we undertake.

Care is an ongoing activity and can help to achieve overall comfort and independence, with the ability for the client to care for themselves. It is important to remember that if a client can care for themselves and have a degree of independence, choice and control, then their overall self-esteem will be high, along with their health and well-being. If we consider these through the eyes of the older person it may give us an insight into what their needs are. These have been divided up into physical and psychological needs, to be fulfilled if the client is to be comfortable.

Physical

Pain
This is the need for pain to be controlled.

Bowel functions
Regular bowel functions need to be monitored, to maintain the client's normal routine.

Disabilities
Consider the loss of function of limbs, hands, eyes, hearing, speech, continence.

Positioning
A suitable position for the client may be in a chair, wheelchair or bed and it is important that the client is assisted into a 'comfortable' position that allows activities to be carried out and full expansion of the lungs.

Consideration needs to be given to the type of chair, foot rests of a wheelchair, the use of cushions/mattress/pillows, the length of time a client may wish to sit out of bed in a chair. Always remembering that the focus of care is the *client* and not the carer's routine. The positioning of the client should be negotiated with the client and the reasons given for the importance of being in one position rather than another. For example, to prevent excess pressure on one part of the body and preventing pressure sores developing.

Psychological

Self-esteem
How is the client feeling:

- Independent
- Worthwhile
- Feeling relaxed and happy with the world
- Having friends and someone to talk to

It has been demonstrated that clients feel more comfortable if they are able to make their own decisions and therefore have more control over their lives and care. It is important that they are given information and the opportunity to discuss treatment and the overall care that is given them.

Rapport with the carers
Friendly relationships with the carers and the feeling of empathy and being cared for are most important for the client. The way in which we communicate with a client can affect the way in which care is given and received (refer to Chapter 2). Clients also need to know who is going to give or assist them with that care and ideally, have a choice of who this should be.

Carers should also be aware of the need for the client to have their own 'personal space' and give the client opportunities to be alone if that is their wish (refer to Chapter 3, Relationships and the Older Person).

Assessment of discomfort

Assessment is undertaken by a professional and the real cause (primary cause) of the discomfort needs to be identified with a holistic approach, by considering physical, cultural, and psychological needs of the client.

The carer can help with the assessment by reporting any observations or any comments made by the client, family or friends (considering the aspects of confidentiality).

This contribution to assessment by the carer complements the ongoing care of the client, and the reporting of the results of any treatment or care given to alleviate discomfort to the person in charge, by verbal or written evaluation of care.

There is no one cause for discomfort and it may be difficult to find the real cause, for instance a client may appear to be very tired. This may be due to pain that prevents sleep, leading to fatigue, anxiety and depression. It is rather like fitting together a jigsaw to try and find the underlying cause of a problem.

Activity 10.13 ■

 Think of the clients you have cared for and list all different ways that you suspected they were in discomfort and pain.

■ ■

Your list may include:

■ Position – curled up, protecting the painful area/limb, muscles become tense
■ Colour – skin may be pale and sweaty, pale face or reddened painful area
■ Rubbing or scratching
■ Respiration and pulse rate – raised
■ Nausea or vomiting – not wishing to eat, anorexia
■ Facial expression – distressed, crying
■ Restless – unable to stay in one position or unable to concentrate, irritable
■ Unable to sleep – leading to fatigue and the inability to 'cope' with the situation
■ Withdrawn and quiet – not wishing to enter into a conversation
■ Aggressive and unco-operative – shouting and demanding care and attention

Pain

Activity 10.14 ■

Consider what can affect the way in which a client perceives pain, write a few notes about a client you care for who has experienced pain.

■ ■

Your notes could include some of the following influences.

Culture

All clients are individuals and will perceive pain differently. Always be aware that not everyone in a particular culture will react in the same way. However, there are some generalizations that can include: suffering in silence an attitude attributed to the British, while others may be more expressive and let it be known they are in pain and discomfort. For example, Eastern Europeans are inclined to be more explicit and openly demonstrate they are in pain.

Previous experiences

Much of our behaviour is coloured by our previous experiences. For instance when we were small if, when we fell over and grazed a knee our mother or guardian was distressed in case there was any bleeding, then in the future should we injure ourselves we would be very concerned. However should the injury in the past be dealt with in a 'matter of fact' way then it may be easier to cope with future injuries.

If, on previous hospital visits the pain and discomfort was dealt with effectively then the client would expect the same on the next visit.

Case study 3

Mr Brown is a diabetic and suffers from pain due to diabetic neuropathy (nerve damage due to diabetes). On his last stay in hospital six months ago he was told 'There is nothing we can do for your pain'. As a result, he feels that he has to accept his pain and does not tell anyone when he is in pain. He is becoming more quiet and withdrawn and the carer just thinks it is his personality and to be expected; so no-one enquires about Mr Brown's comfort or reports his change in condition to the person in charge.

However we must always remember a quote from McCaffery (a writer on pain) 'Pain is what the client says it is and exists when he says it does' (McCaffery, 1983). The concept of pain is different from the client to client and we must always take the client's perception/understanding of pain and act upon it. Pain is a private and multi-dimensional experience, meaning that it affects various parts of our body, mind and senses.

Carers have their own perception of what pain a client is experiencing and therefore may feel the client is 'over-reacting, just enjoying the attention or the effect of the analgesic'. As a result, the carer takes a punitive and judgemental view, both of the client and the amount of pain and discomfort they are experiencing. Consequently they do not report the pain and discomfort to the person in charge straight away, thus preventing the client receiving the care and attention they need.

Pain can be measured by various pain assessment tools, some are a scale 1–10 and the client puts a dot or indicates where on the scale their current level of pain is.

NO PAIN ◄————————————————► A LOT OF PAIN
0   1   2   3   4   5   6   7   8   9   10

In the case of a young child, faces can be used, a happy smiling one for no pain and an unhappy crying face for a lot of pain.

Some clients may be unable to communicate easily and convey the intensity or the location of the pain as they may have a language barrier, suffering from or be brain damage due to a stroke or confusion. But just because a client cannot verbalize the amount of pain they are suffering does not mean they do not feel pain.

Pain can be difficult to assess in the older person, especially those suffering from Alzheimer's Disease (where the client suffers from dementia with loss of short-term memory and has difficulty in expressing themselves). It has been shown that in one incident a client suffering from severe Alzheimer's did not receive any analgesics following a below the knee amputation. It is sometimes the case that if a client does not complain of pain they do not receive any analgesics (painkillers).

It is the role of the carer to report any signs that a client is in pain and always to be receptive to both the client's and the relatives' needs. The person in charge should always discuss pain control with the client and also inform family and friends that the client's pain can be controlled or relieved by a variety of methods.

Treatment of pain

Relieving the client's pain decreases their suffering and will help them to cope with other stresses. For example, removing a chronic pain, postoperative pain or the pain suffered from shingles will enable a client to think, participate in treatment, such as breathing exercises and also plan for the future.

The principles of relieving pain include the following:

- Is your client in pain?
- What have they used before?
- What do *they* think will work?
- What is the client willing to try?

Try it; evaluate the effect, did it relieve the pain? Report back to the person in charge and ensure records are completed.

Activity 10.15 ■■■■■■■■■■■■■■■■■■■■■■■■■■

 Can you list the various methods used for pain relief?

■■■■■■■■■■■■■■■■■■■■■■■■■■■■■

Your list may include:

- Change the position of the client
- Neurosurgical techniques
- Analgesics (pain killers)
- Reduce anxiety
- Diversion/distraction
- Support relatives and friends
- Apply heat/cold
- Acupuncture

- Antinflammatory tablets/creams
- Information, explanation, allow choices and alternatives
- Relaxation
- Massage
- Reflexology
- Imagery
- Rest

General care for clients in pain

Direct care

A variety of methods can be used to alleviate pain.

Position
Support with pillows and frequent changes of position can aid mobility and prevent pressure sores.

Exercise
Active and passive movements will reduce muscle tension.

Bed
Ensure it is free from wrinkles, supportive mattress, loose bed clothes to give comfort and aid movement.

Chair
The chair or wheelchair must be the correct height, use a foot rest if required to help comfortable position and support.

Indirect care

Environment
Remove excess stimuli from the environment such as bright lights, loud sudden noises, inadequate heating or ventilation, or untidy surroundings.

Replace them with dimmed lights, fresh air at a suitable temperature for the client and familiar belongings, such as photographs, plants and furniture to increase feeling of security.

Specific care

No one treatment or routine will be suitable for all clients and often different types will be used to help the client. Each one is an individual with different needs.

Medication

Analgesics can be given by different routes and can be given intermittently or continually. One method of managing post-operative and terminal illness pain is allowing the patient to control the painkiller; patient-controlled analgesia. This method removes the peaks of sedation and troughs of pain, by the client controlling the amount of analgesic injected into a vein from a syringe pump.

It is thought that those with an extrovert type of personality will complain and let others know they are in pain, thereby receiving regular analgesic cover. The quiet, introverted person on the other hand, will not receive adequate analgesics as 'they do not like to complain' and will suffer in silence.

Tranquillisers, and sedation will reduce anxiety and also help the client to sleep.

Different diversions may also be used which would help to distract the client from thinking about the pain.

Therapeutic touch, massage

This is a form of touch that can communicate messages from one person to another. It has a relaxing effect on the client, as it increases the flexibility of muscles and blood flow. The increase in the circulation and venous return helps to remove waste products from the tissues and helps to prevent contractures of muscles and tension.

It can be very therapeutic to massage a client's hands, feet or back. Just the fact that you are spending time to be with the client has a positive effect. In one study (Jones in the Observer © 1994), it was found that aromas and massage had an extremely beneficial effect on clients with Alzheimer's Disease by reducing the effects of confusion and 'easing the pains on old age'.

Note: always check that the use of massage is included in the clients' plan of care and that you are competent to undertake it.

Relaxation

There are simple relaxation techniques that once learned and used can be very effective and help the client to be in control, as they can undertake relaxation exercises when they wish to. Any exercise should be written on the client's plan of care (refer to Chapter 13, Caring for Carers).

Music

The use of a personal stereo and headphones will enable a client to listen to the music of their choice. Try to find out what the clients' preferences are. Listening to favourite and familiar music may help the client to relax and bring back happy memories and associations of the past.

Taped stories are also helpful, as the client can get quite absorbed in an exciting tale and forget their discomfort.

Visualization/imagery

This can be achieved with the use of music or a tape and someone describing a beautiful scene walking along a beach, river or in the countryside. This calming and relaxing explanation can help to reduce stress and anxiety and enable the client to 'cope' with pain more effectively.

Aromatherapy

This is the use of oils, which have a relaxing effect on the client. They can be used in vaporizers, body massage, added to the bath or in compress. Care should be taken to check the suitability of the use of aromatherapy for each client, because aromatherapy can have an adverse effect on the client who is taking some types of medication or suffering from certain illnesses. Studies have found that aromatherapy is beneficial for clients suffering from Alzheimer's Disease, (Jones in *Observer* © 1994)

Note: always check that the use of aromatherapy is included in the clients' plan of care and that you are competent to undertake it.

Acupuncture

This specialist procedure consists of the insertion of small needles in specific places with the effect of reducing pain.

Transcutaneous electrical stimulation (TENS)

Two small pads are attached to the skin and a small electrical current is passed through them. Pain can be reduced without the treatment having any adverse effect on the client (Fig. 10.7).

It can be used for the client with chronic pain, such as rheumatoid arthritis or an amputee with phantom limb pain.

Fig. 10.7 Client
receiving TENS treatment.

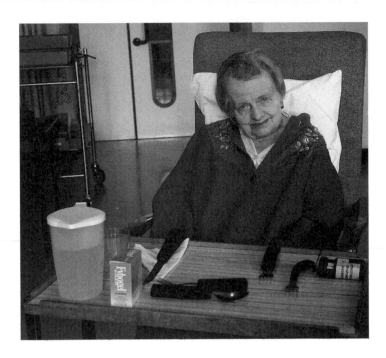

Sleep and rest

Sleep is thought to be restorative and the time for our bodies and brain to rest. The amount of sleep we need changes with each individual and throughout our lives. The changes that occur in the older person include:

■ A decrease in total sleep time, although the time spent in bed may be longer
■ A slight increase in sleep time after the age of 80
■ Taking a longer time to get off to sleep
■ Disturbed sleep with frequent wakenings after the age of 50

Adapted from Pascal & Woodhouse (1994).

Activity 10.16 ■

 Make a list of what disturbs your sleep.

■ ■

The list could be endless and in the older person, especially in females there is an increased incidence of insomnia. Insomnia means disturbed sleep with a reduced quality or quantity of sleep and frequently it can lead to tiredness and a feeling of being moody and depressed the next day (Jago, 1995).

Causes of insomnia in the older person can include:

- Bladder problems
- Chronic pain
- Cough
- Bereavement, following a bereavement insomnia can last up to four years
- Mood changes, e.g. anxiety or depression
- Dementia
- Drugs, e.g. caffeine (found in coffee and tea) alcohol and some 'heart drugs' (beta blockers)

For further details see Jago (1995).

A patient with rheumatoid arthritis can have an interrupted sleep pattern, even when they are not experiencing a flare-up and joints are not painful. This may be due to a habit that has been set up when joints are painful and they find it difficult to get comfortable in bed, and sleep becomes fragmented.

Sleeplessness is a client's problem that carers can help to solve.

Activity 10.17 ■■■■■■■■■■■■■■■■■■■■■■■■■■■■■

How can you provide an environment that would promote sleep?

■■■■■■■■■■■■■■■■■■■■■■■■■■■■■■■

You may have thought of:

- Quietness, hushed voices, absence of squeaky doors, wheels, etc. (the older person is more sensitive to noise)
- Subdued lighting, but with a light switch near to the client
- Good ventilation with a temperature of 21°C
- Light but warm night and bed clothes
- 'Being around for the client' and a call system to hand

Activity 10.18 ■■■■■■■■■■■■■■■■■■■■■■■■■■■■

List aspects of *physical care* that would encourage sleep.

■■■■■■■■■■■■■■■■■■■■■■■■■■■■■■■

Your list could include:

- Emptying the bladder
- Controlling pain
- Position well supported with pillows should the client have difficulty with breathing or complain of indigestion
- Avoid stimulants such as caffeine and nicotine, avoid large meals. Although alcohol is sometimes helpful to initiate sleep, it tends to disrupt it later in the night
- Milky drink
- Physical and mental activity should be encouraged during the day, but avoid anything too strenuous before bedtime

- Massage or a relaxing bath before bedtime
- Do not sleep during the day
- The use of a hypnotic drug (sleeping tablet) may be prescribed ideally for short periods only, any repeat prescriptions should be carefully reviewed and any adverse effects monitored

Medication

All clients receiving night sedation should be monitored for any adverse signs due to residual effect of the drug. These may include, difficulty in waking up or appearing drowsy and being unsteady on their feet, with the possibility of falls in the morning.

It is a fact that 30% of the residents in residential homes use hypnotic drugs on a regular basis. Some of the older type of drugs (benzodiazepine) have been associated with adverse effects and, particularly with the longer acting medications, residual hangover effects the following day. More modern night sedation starts working very quickly and causes no problems with concentration or alertness the following day.

All clients taking night sedation should be observed for any signs of confusion, drowsiness or appearing to be unsteady on their feet. Should any of these signs be evident the person in charge, or the doctor should be informed immediately. It may indicate an adverse reaction to the night sedation that the client is receiving. This may be an indication that the client needs to change their current medication.

Activity 10.19 ■

List the *psychological* aspects that could promote sleep

■ ■

The following could be of help to the client:

- Develop a routine and sleep pattern, save sleep for night-time and only go to bed when feeling tired, try to get up at the same time each morning. The use of a sleep diary may be of help to establish clients' sleeping habits (SLEEPtalk, 1995).
- If it is difficult to get to sleep, get up or do something relaxing and then try to get off to sleep.
- Solve any problems before trying to go to sleep.
- Allow visitors, or a pet to stay with the client until they are asleep.

It is important to find out what the client's normal sleep pattern is and their routine before going to sleep. We should try to accommodate the client in order to keep to his or her usual routine. For instance, reading or listening to music may be part of the normal routine, or watching television. This may result in some form of compromise should the client share a room with someone who has a different routine and wishes to go to sleep earlier. Sleep patterns and any routines should be included in the care plan, which should be frequently evaluated and updated.

Summary

In this chapter we have considered the overall comfort of the client including the definition of comfort and what it means to the older person. The way in which hygiene needs can be met and the holistic and individualized aspects of care are discussed. The causes and the prevention of pressure sores are clarified emphasizing the importance of their prevention. This chapter also explains the various ways in which the clients' pain can be relieved and how the carer can help to promote sleep and rest in the older person.

References

Blicharz (1979) in *Current practice in Nursing Care of the Adult*. Edited by Kennedy, M. & Pfeifer, G., CV Mosby Co., London.

Fairclough, A. (1993) Please call the dentist. *Elderly Care*, October/November **5** (5), 23.

Goodwin, S. (1994) Personal laundry: an essential part of patient care. *Nursing Times*, 27 July **90** (30), 31.

Jago, W. (1995) Does insomnia matter in older people? *Geriatric Medicine*, May, 12–15.

Jones, J. in Observer © (1994) Aromas and massage to ease the pains of age. *The Guardian, Health Supplement*, 16 August.

McCaffery, M. (1983) *Nursing the Patient in Pain*. Harper and Row, London.

McMahon, C. & Harding, J. (1994) *Knowledge to Care. A Handbook For Care Assistants*, Blackwell Science, Oxford.

Pascal, J. & Woodhouse, K. (1994) The effective management of insomnia. *Geriatric Medicine*, February, 41–44.

SLEEPtalk (1995) *Getting Back to Sleep* and *Getting a Good Nights Sleep* Leaflets available from Lorex, Luna House, Field House Lane, Globe Park, Marlow, Bucks SL7 1LW.

Further reading

Booth, R. (1994) Keeping in touch. *Nursing Times*, 2 November **90** (44), 29.

Campbell, J. (1994) Skin deep. *Nursing Times*, 23 February, **90** (8), 50.

Clements, D., Ryan, A. & Lowry, R. (1994) Pressure sore prevention. *Nursing Times*, 24 April, **90** (24), 20 and 69.

Fox, P. & Delve, M. (1994) Equipped to care. *Nursing Times*, 27 July, **90** (30), 46.

Hudson, R. (1994) Lavender oils relaxation in older patients. *Nursing Times*, 27 July, **90** (30), 12.

Lyons, Y. (1994) Monitoring practice. *Nursing Times*, 20 April, **90** (16), 69.

Mason, P. (1994) Pain relief. *Nursing Times*, 31 August, **90** (35), 24.

Matlhoko, D. (1994) Surface tension. *Nursing Times*, 19 January, **90** (3), 60. November, **90** (47), 42.

McDonald, S. (1994) Controlled environment. *Nursing Times*, 23.

Mullineaux, J. (1994) Delays increase risk of pressure sores in A&E. *Nursing Times*, 26 January **90** (4), 11.

Parsons, G. (1994) The benefits of relaxation in the control of pain. *Nursing Times*, 11 May, **90** (19), 11.

Reid, J. & Morison M. (1994) Classification of pressure sores, *Nursing Times*, 18 May, **90** (20), 46.

Trevalyan, J. & Booth, B. (1994) Aromatherapy, Complementary Medicine Supplement. *Nursing Times*, 21 September **90** (38), 3.

Walding, M. (1994) Skin treatment. *Nursing Times*, 16 February **90** (7), 78.

Wherry, C. (1994) Private enterprise (patient privacy). *Nursing Times*, 26 January, **90**, 52.

Hygiene

Davis, L. (1994) *Social Care for Elderly People*. Available from Social Care Association (Educ.) Wrentham House, 23 Queens Road, Coventry CV1 3EG.

Help the Aged (1994) *Giving Good care, An Introductory Guide For Care Assistants*. Available free from Help the Aged, St James Walk, Clerkenwell Green, London EC1R 0BE.

Jenkins, G. (1993) Rough and tumble, guide to laundering. *Elderly Care*, January/February, **6** (1), 14.

Nazarko, L. (1996) Chapter 11 in *NVQs in Nursing and Residential Homes*, Blackwell Science, Oxford.

Comfort

Benbow, M. (1993) Better than cure. *Nursing Times*, 25 August, **89** (34), 55.

Birchall, L. (1993) Making sense of pressure sore prediction calculators. *Nursing Times*, 5 May **89** (18), 34.

Booth, B. (1993) Therapeutic touch. *Nursing Times*, 4 August **89** (31), 48.

Booth, B. (1993) Soft options. *Nursing Times*, 25 August **89** (34), 60.

Chaitow, L. (1993) *The Book of Pain Relief*. Thorsons, an Imprint of Harper Collins Publishers, London.

Closs, S. (1993) Malnutrition: the key to pressure sores. *Nursing Standard*, 25 January, **8**, (4), 32.

East, E. (1992) How much does it hurt? *Nursing Times*, 30 Septermber **88** (40), 48–9.

Fascione, J. (1995) Healing power of touch. *Elderly Care*, January/February, **7** (1), 19.

Partridge, C. (1994) Pain in confused patients. *Elderly Care*, September/October, **6** (5), 19.

Prkachin, K. (1993) Facial expressions as pain indicators. *Nursing Times*, 14 April **89** (15), 58.

Rigby, W. (1995) *Natural therapies for older people*. Hawker, London.

Scruttons, S. (1993) *Ageing Healthily and in Control*, Chapman & Hall, London.

Seymour, J. (1995) Pain control, TENS machines. *Nursing Times*, 8 February, **91** (6), 51.

Sofaer, B. (1984) *Pain: a Handbook for Nurses*. Harper & Row, London.

Swiatczak, L (1992) Choice thoughts. *Elderly Care*, July/August **4** (4), 40.

Trevelyan, J. (1993) Aromatherapy. *Nursing Times*, 23 June, **89** (25), 38.

Trevelyan, J. (1993) Fringe benefits. *Nursing Times*, 28 April, **89** (17), 30.

Trevelyan, J. (1993) Massage. *Nursing Times*, 12 May, **89** (19), 45.

Tutton, E. (1991) Chapter 7, Massage in nursing, in *Nursing as a Therapy*. McMahon, R. & Pearson, A. (Eds) Chapman & Hall, London.

West, B. (1994) The essence of aromatherapy. *Elderly Care*, September/October, **6** (5), 21.

Rest

Dias, B. (1992) Things that go bump in the night. *Nursing Times*, 16 September, **88** (38), 36–38.

Grace, J. (1994) Hypnotics in general practice. *Geriatric Medicine*, May, 35–39.

Horne, L.A. (1991) No more wakeful nights: helping elderly people to sleep properly. *Professional Nurse*, April, **6** (7), 383.

Willis, J. (1989) A good night's sleep. *Nursing Times*, 22 November, **88** (47), 29–31.

Useful addresses

E45 Self Help Leaflets
PO Box 12,
West PDO
Lenton
Nottingham NG7 2GB
Information concerning Over 60s Skin Care, Common Rashes and Itchy Skin, Dry and Uncomfortable Skin. Please send A5 SAE.

Social Care Association (Education)
Wrentham House
23 Queens Road
Coventry CV1 3EG
Code of Practice for social care, information booklet *Giving Good Care*.

The British Foot Wear Manufacturers
Royalty House
72 Dean Street
London W1V 5HB

Bury Boot and Shoe Company
Northampton

The Society of Chiropodists
53 Welbeck Street
London W1M 7HE

The Pain Relief Foundation
Rice Lane
Liverpool, L9 1AE
Information concerning, coping with chronic pain, to include back, phantom limb, facial, cancer, diabetes and shingles pain. Please send SAE, (A4 size and 36p stamp)

Cancer Relief
Macmillan Nurses
Anchor House
15–19 Britten Street
London SW3 3TY

The Institute of Complementary Medicine
4, Tavern Quay
Plough Way
London SE16 1QZ

SLEEPtalk
Healthfacts
PO Box 2353
London W8 6ZT. Send SAE.

Chapter 11
Mobility and Safer Client Handling
Susan Fell

Overview

Mobility refers to the ability of an individual to move independently through life space. Loss of mobility is a common problem for ageing persons. The reasons for this are explored in the chapter and ways to promote and improve mobility are discussed.

The chapter highlights:

- The responsibilities of the employer and employee under The Health and Safety at Work Act 1974 (Health and Safety Commission, 1974) and the Manual Handling Operations Regulations 1992 (Health and Safety Commission, 1992)
- The principles of safer lifting and the problems associated with top heavy movements are explained
- Ways in which the carer can assist the client to move when they are unable to do so independently

Carers undertaking manual handling of a client should receive training accompanied by supervised practice. The chapter gives guidance to reinforce what has already been taught.

Key words

Legislation, risk assessment, care plan, communication, weight bear, stand, passive/active exercises, muscle tone.

What is mobility?

Everyday activities such as eating and drinking, eliminating, washing and dressing, involve movement. Independence is impossible without some degree of mobility.

Mobility describes the capacity for movement. It involves the work of large muscles such as those that enable you to stand, sit, walk and run. Movement is made possible by the contraction and relaxation of muscles under the control of the nervous system. In healthy people all muscles are in a state of muscle tone. Muscle strength declines with age and muscles which are used infrequently lose tone, becoming wasted.

Mobility may be restricted temporarily or permanently. The causes of immobility include physical, psychological and environmental factors.

Physical factors effecting mobility

An individual's mobility and independence are reliant on the normal functioning of the nervous, musculoskeletal, respiratory, and circulatory systems. Injury or disease to one or more of these systems may lead to difficulty with mobility.

Physical Symptom	Example of possible underlying condition
Breathlessness	chronic obstructive airways disease (COAD) congestive cardiac failure (CCF) lung cancer (Ca lung)
Pain	osteo/rheumatoid arthritis following surgery cancer bone metastases
Angina	cardiac failure hypertension (high blood pressure)
Instability	cerebral-vascular accident (CVA) Parkinson's disease
Visual impairment	cataracts

Psychological factors

These include

- Anxiety
- Depression
- Fear of falling
- Forgetfulness
- Fear of being attacked
- Nowhere to go to
- No-one to go with

Environmental factors

These include

- Uneven floor surfaces
- Difficult access (stairs, steep ramp)
- Not enough space

Do you know?

Fear of falling is common in elderly persons, more so in women than men. It is associated with decreased quality of life, increased frailty, and recent experience of falls. (Arfren *et al.*, 1994)

Immobility can lead to further complications such as oedema, pressure sores and subsequent pain. If the causes of immobility can be treated, further deterioration may be reduced or prevented (refer to Chapter 10, Comfort and Rest.)

Remember if you don't use it you lose it!

Many clients admitted to hospitals, nursing and residential homes regain lost function by their own efforts, or as a result of recovering from the disease that caused them to be less mobile.

The aim of rehabilitation is not just what the client does whilst in hospital, but what they do and continue to do at home. Home visits are of great importance prior to discharge from hospital (refer to Chapter 7, Supported Living). Psychological and environmental barriers to mobility which may not have been evident in the hospital setting can then be identified. Recommendations can be made including changes in the position of furniture; provision of aids; fitting of handrails; the provision of downstairs toilet and hygiene facilities; the conversion of a bathroom to a walk/wheel-in shower room; the installation of overhead tracking systems, etc.

Health and safety legislation

Health and Safety at Work etc. Act 1974 (HSAWA 1974)

Under the HASAWA 1974 all employers have a general duty to take all reasonably practicable steps to ensure the health, safety and welfare of their employees.

This includes:

- The provision and maintenance of equipment and safe systems of work
- The provision of information, instruction, supervision and training
- Arrangements for the safe transport and storage of equipment including ease of access to and from the work area

The Manual Handling Operations Regulations 1992 (MHOR 1992)

Under the MHOR 1992 a 'load' includes inanimate or animate objects. 'Manual handling operations' refers to the transporting or supporting of a load (including the lifting, putting down, pushing, pulling, carrying or moving thereof) by hand or bodily force.

Employer's responsibilities

Each employer shall avoid the need for his or her employees to carry out manual handling tasks which involve a risk of them being injured. Where such handling cannot be avoided a risk assessment must be carried out taking into account the following five factors:

(1) The task
(2) The load
(3) The environment
(4) Individual capability
(5) Other factors e.g. personal protective clothing (uniform)

The employer must also take steps to remove or reduce the risk of injury to the lowest level that is reasonably practicable using the assessment as a basis for action.

The HASAWA 1974 and the MHOR 1992 also contain responsibilities for employees. The employee is required to:

- Co-operate with the employer in making full and proper use of equipment provided
- Take opportunities they are given in relation to training
- Take reasonable care of their own health and safety and that of others who may be affected by their activities.
- Report to their employer any health problems they have that could affect their capability

Activity 11.1 ■

Find and read the manual handling policy for your area.

■ ■

Reporting of Injuries, Diseases and Dangerous Occurrences Regulations 1985 (RIDDOR 1985)

If you are involved in an accident/incident relating to manual handling inform the person in charge of your area. An incident form must be completed following any adverse incident that occurs in the work place. The incident can then be investigated and action taken to prevent or reduce the risk of it happening again.

Depending on the severity of the injury sustained or the length of time you are off sick (three days or more), the incident may need to be reported by your employer to the Health and Safety Executive (HSE).

Activity 11.2 ■

What are the procedures for reporting accidents/incidents in your area? Can you think of an accident/incident that occurred while moving a client in your work place, what were the consequences? Could the incident have been prevented?
How?

■ ■

Manual handling risk assessment

Under health and safety legislation if a client needs help to move, a manual handling risk assessment must be completed by a trained member of staff, and referred to before any attempt is made to move them.

AREA OF ASSESSMENT	YES	NO	EXAMPLE OF CHANGES THAT COULD BE MADE
Task Where is the client to be moved to?			
Does it involve: holding or supporting the client away from the trunk? twisting and rotating the spine? stooping?			Could a different technique be used to bring you closer to the client
handling the client above your chest height?			Could the height of the surface you are transferring the client from/to, be adjusted to assist in the activity
handling the client below your knee level?			
excessive lifting and lowering distances?			
strenuous pushing and pulling?			
Working environment Are there: space constraints preventing good posture?			Could furniture be removed, rearranged
poor floors i.e. slippery, uneven, unstable?			Could floor surfaces be changed (e.g. remove rugs; linoleum flooring rather than carpet)
variations in levels of floor or surfaces (slopes, steps)?			Provide ramps rather than steps
poor lighting conditions?			Could lighting be improved
Hot, cold, humid conditions?			
Does equipment take up space?			Would overhead tracking be preferable to a mobile hoist?

AREA OF ASSESSMENT	YES	NO	EXAMPLE OF CHANGES THAT COULD BE MADE
Individual capability of the Carer Does the job: require unusual strength?			Could the task be mechanized
create a hazard for those with a health problem e.g. back pain, joint pain?			
create a hazard for those who are pregnant?			
call for special instruction, information and training for safer performance of the task; are you competent to carry out the task?			Could information and training be given?
require two or more people to carry out the task safely?			
Other factors Is your movement/posture restricted by the clothing worn?			Could a style of dress be worn that does not hinder movement
Load			This would be the client (see below)

THE CLIENT

Name . . . .

Age . . . . Height . . . .

Weight . . . . Sex . . . .

ASSESSMENT	YES	NO	COMMENT
Co-operative?			
Understand simple instructions?			
History of dizziness or falls?			
Able to stand?			

ASSESSMENT	YES	NO	COMMENT
Able to walk? If yes, how far? Able to climb stairs? If yes, how many?			
Able to maintain a sitting position?			
Able to move up in bed?			
Able to get: in/out of bed? in/out of a chair? on/off the toilet? in/out of a bath?			
Is able to grip with both hands?			
Does the client normally use aids?			
Handling constraints: Pain? Skin condition? Infusions/attachments? Other?			

CLIENT TO BE MOVED IN THE FOLLOWING WAY:

MOVE	EQUIPMENT	No of STAFF	PROCEDURE TO FOLLOW

Signature: Status   Date   Review Date

Once the assessment has been completed the most appropriate method of assisting the client to move should be decided, using a multi-disciplinary approach. The initial assessment must be reviewed regularly, or when changes occur in the client's condition, or any other area in relation to the assessment changes.

Activity 11.3 ■■■■■■■■■■■■■■■■■■■■■■■■■■■■■■

 Look at your clients' assessment and care plans, is there sufficient information available to enable you to move them safety?

■■■■■■■■■■■■■■■■■■■■■■■■■■■■■■■■■■■

Posture and safer handling

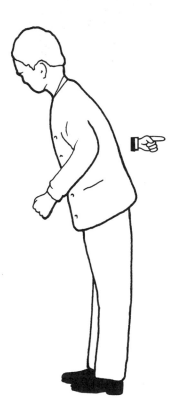

Fig. 11.1 Stooped posture.

The top heavy posture (stooping)

This is a posture that many of us adopt during our daily activities: using a vacuum cleaner, ironing, washing up, brushing teeth, making a bed, picking a piece of paper up from the floor (Fig. 11.1).

Activity 11.4 ■■■■■■■■■■■■■■■■■■■■■■■■■■■■

Observe at work and at home activities that result in stooping. Is it always necessary or could it be avoided?

■■■■■■■■■■■■■■■■■■■■■■■■■■■■■■■■■■

The top heavy posture causes:

(1) Excessive work of the back muscles to prevent us from falling forwards.
(2) Reduced skill and efficiency. If all efforts are focused on preventing us from falling, what efforts are left for the task in hand?
(3) Progressive loss of normal tissue elasticity. This would occur as a result of restricted blood flow to the back muscles during static loading.
(4) Excessive use of purely muscular effort. Imagine performing a tug of war in this position. All the work would be done by your arm muscles as the posture does not allow you to transfer body weight from one leg to the other as in Fig. 11.2.

Activity 11.5 ■■■■■■■■■■■■■■■■■■■■■■■■■■■■■

 Place one foot in front of the other, make a fairly wide base and practise transferring your body weight forward over the front leg and then back

■■■■■■■■■■■■■■■■■■■■■■■■■■■■■■■■■■■

For movement to be efficient it must achieve its objective with the minimum of muscle effort, and the minimum of cumulative strain. The

Fig. 11.2 Weight transfer.

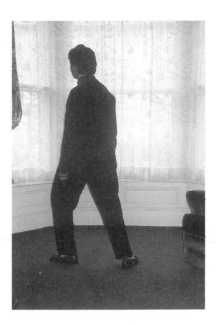 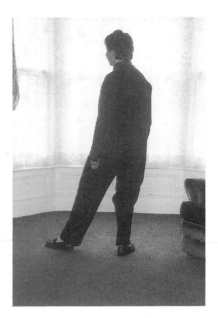

posture adopted by the carer at the start of any client handling procedure is of vital importance. If the initial posture is top heavy, threat to loss of balance will produce unnecessary muscle stiffening.

The top heavy posture can be avoided by sitting down to perform a task; raising the bed to a more suitable level to make it; kneeling on the floor to perform a task; or bending your knees rather than your back to pick up something up from the floor.

Do you know?

 Wearing gardener's knee pads is a useful way of reminding you to kneel rather than stoop and they are very comfortable too.

Principles of safer client handling techniques

- Get as close to the client as you can.
- Keep your back naturally erect and your head up.
- Make sure you have a wide stable base.
- Ensure knees are slightly flexed and not locked. This may be a position that allows you to transfer your weight from front leg to back leg, from side to side or by bending your knees from a higher level to a lower level and vice versa.
- Ensure you have a secure hold on the client.
- Avoid twisting.
- Use your strong thigh muscles to bring about the movement of the client.

Caring for the carer

All manual handling particularly of clients is inherently unsafe. When a client is moved manually, all those involved are potentially at risk of injury. The client may be injured, experience pain or discomfort due to being moved in an unsafe or unsuitable fashion. The carer may be injured by attempting to move a client beyond his or her capabilities. The importance of a detailed assessment has already been discussed. All situations must be assessed individually by a trained person.

It is unsafe and unacceptable for two carers to take the full weight of a client when moving them. There is equipment available that enables clients to be moved by:

- Sliding the client using friction-free surfaces
- Lifting the client using a hoist

Injuries that may be sustained through postural stress and the lifting of heavy loads (clients) include the following.

Strained back muscles

The back muscles are not designed to lift heavy loads. They are for maintaining posture and allowing flexibility and range of movement. Beware any task that requires flexion or twisting of the spine when moving a load.

Strained/torn ligaments in the back

This is very common and can be extremely painful. The ligaments are likely to be overstretched and strained when postures are adopted which cause the individual to be more than 45° out of the vertical. These ligaments are also more susceptible to injury during and following pregnancy.

Prolapsed/slipped discs

The intervertebral discs are positioned between the vertebra. They are filled with fluid to enable them to act as shock absorbers and help to dissipate the forces put on the spine. During the course of the day we become about 1 cm shorter. This is due to pressures placed on the spine and the forces of gravity causing some of the fluid to be expelled from the discs. If we don't have sufficient time to rest and recover from a day's activity, approximately eight hours lying down over a 24 hour period, the spine is going to be more prone to injury. The discs in this instance may begin to degenerate putting pressure on the facet joints. The continual wear and tear of the disc may cause weakened areas in the annulus through which the nucleus may prolapse. The prolapsed disc can exert pressure on one of the nerves from the spinal cord, resulting in referred pain e.g. sciatica. This is pain felt in the buttock, down the leg and sometimes in the foot, due to pressure being placed on the sciatic nerve where it exits the lumbar spine (Fig. 11.3).

Fig. 11.3 The spine.

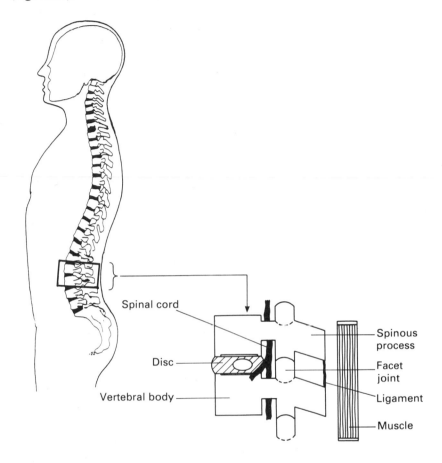

Do you know?

One in four health care workers experiences back ache at the end of their working day. (COSHE, 1992).
Between 1992 and 1993, 93.16 million working days were lost due to certified sickness for back pain (Department of Social Security, 1994).

If you do have an aching back

(1) Seek the advice of your GP or visit your occupational health department. You may also obtain useful advice from the National Back Pain Association.
(2) Avoid lifting.
(3) Ensure you have adequate rest and recovery time between performing tasks.

At the end of the day rather than slumping into a low sofa (creating poor posture and giving little support to your back) try one of the following methods:

- Lie on the floor on your front. Bring your elbows forward and raise the top part of your body supporting it on your forearms – an ideal position for reading a book, or watching television (this position provides an opportunity to stretch the back out of the stooped posture).
- Lie flat on your back on the floor with a firm support under your head. Raise your lower legs up on a chair creating a right angle at the hip and knee joints (Fig. 11.4). Put on your favourite most relaxing piece of music and rest for 10–20 minutes (this position keeps the spine in alignment and reduces the compressive forces put on it).

Fig. 11.4 Relaxing the spine after a hard day's work.

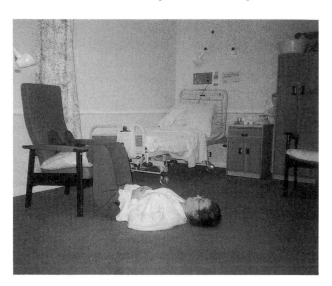

If you find either of the above uncomfortable then do not continue. Try to find time to relax in a position that is comfortable for you.

Remember, if you are caring for someone else you need to take care of yourself. Exercises such as swimming and walking help you to relax as well as stay fit.

Activity 11.6 ■

 Find your favourite most relaxing piece of music; lie down and relax!

■ ■

Exercise in the elderly

Exercise in the elderly is an essential component to help maintain mobility and health. Exercise will help promote joint motion and muscle strength, stimulate circulation and prevent contractures.

Exercises can be performed independently by the client (active), with the help of the carer (active assisted), or by the carer with no active involvement of the client (passive).

Clients should be encouraged to put all joints through a full range of movement at least once a day. These can be demonstrated and taught to the carer/client by the physiotherapist.

If the carer needs to assist with these exercises the following points should be remembered:

- Offer support above and below the joint being exercised.
- Exercise the joint at least three times moving it smoothly and slowly.
- Do not force the joint if there is resistance or pain.

A range of motion exercises for the foot will increase circulation and mobility in the legs and feet (Fig. 11.5).

Fig. 11.5 Foot exercises.

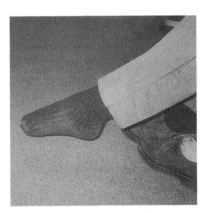 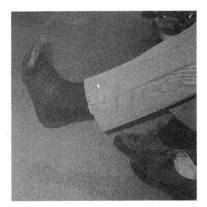

Do you know?

Low intensity resistance weight training of the lower extremities can lead to significant gains in muscle strength and can affect the functional mobility of healthy independent older adults up to the age of 93 years. (Noble *et al.*, 1994)

Proper positioning of the client

Comfort, breathing, circulation and prevention of complications such as contractures, can be facilitated by correct body alignment. If the client is unable to do this unaided it can be performed by the carer (Fig. 11.6).

Fig. 11.6 (a) client slumping in chair (b) client sitting correctly.

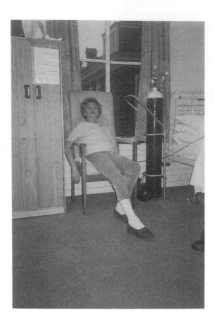 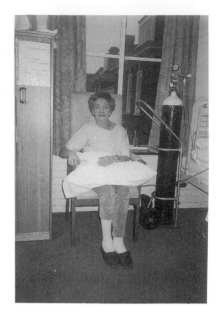

Activity 11.7 ■■■■■■■■■■■■■■■■■■■■■■■■■■■■■

 Observe the clients in your care. Are they in the optimal position? Seek advice from nursing or care staff, physiotherapist, occupational therapist.

■■■■■■■■■■■■■■■■■■■■■■■■■■■■■■■■■

Client handling techniques

This section of the chapter gives step by step guidelines to enable the carer to have an understanding of a variety of manual handling techniques. In order to do this the client mobility assessment sheet will be examined closely.

The handling technique to be performed and equipment that may be required must be discussed with the client prior to its use. This will give the client and carer the opportunity to express any concerns they may have regarding the above.

Co-operation

A client should not be physically forced to move. This would not only put the client at risk of injury but also the carer. If a client actively resists when you attempt to move them stop and question why?

- Do they need to move?
- Do they want to move?
- Are they in pain?
- Are they afraid?
- Is the method appropriate?

Some clients may be quite happy to get out of bed after 10.00 AM but not before. Any attempt to try could result in a completely wasted effort. If you are uncertain of how to proceed in a situation stop and seek advice.

Understanding simple instructions

Ensure your client has an understanding of how you are going to assist them and what you require them to do. In order for this communication to be effective, the following should be considered:

- Ensure the client can see and hear you while you speak. Speak clearly and concisely using language appropriate for them.
- If appropriate, ensure the client is wearing their glasses or has their hearing aid switched on.
- Check that they have understood your explanation.
- If equipment is to be used you may wish to show pictures or demonstrate it on a colleague.
- Plan ahead. Don't wait until the client urgently needs the toilet then explain for the first time how you will assist them to stand.

History of dizziness or falls

The reason for this would need to be discovered; possible causes may be:

- Poor lighting
- Loose carpets
- Relying on unstable furniture
- Walking too far
- Unsuitable aids
- Medication

These may have been identified in the environmental assessment however, there may be other reasons. For example the client may suffer from postural hypotension, i.e. the client's blood pressure drops causing them to feel dizzy and unbalanced when they stand. This situation may be resolved by assisting the client to stand in stages e.g. bed-standing:

- The client sits up in bed; allow time for them to adjust to the change of posture.
- The client sits on the edge of the bed for a few moments, again giving time for the cardiovascular system to adapt to the change in position.
- The client stands.

Further assessment of client's history of falls may indicate they should not actually be walking, or the distance they are trying to walk is beyond their capability.

Able to weight bear

Is the client able to take weight through their legs? Factors which will affect a client's ability to weight bear include:

- Pain
- Fracture of a lower limb e.g. femur.
- Orthopaedic surgery to a lower limb e.g. uncemented total hip replacement.

Able to stand

Some clients may be able to take weight through their limbs but due to poor muscle tone are unable to get into or maintain the standing position.

Able to walk

If the client is able to weight bear through both legs and able to stand, it is likely that they will be able to walk.

Clients who can stand and weight bear through one leg only may be able to walk with the aid of crutches, or a Zimmer frame.

Once the ability of the client to walk is known then the distance they can walk needs to be clarified. The distance may be affected by: fatigue, breathlessness or pain.

It may be that the distance a client can walk can be improved upon, but never try to walk a client beyond their capability. This may result in a fall that could then cause the client to lose much of their confidence.

Before assisting a client to walk ensure the environment is clear of obstructions with good lighting. One or two chairs could be positioned along the distance to be covered in case the client tires. The client should be appropriately dressed, i.e. in clothes that fit correctly and allow ease of movement without the risk of the clothes falling down. It is not easy to walk while trying to hold up a pair of pyjamas three sizes too big! Footwear should be comfortable and well fitting.

Equipment is often used by a client that enables them to walk independently. This may be a handrail on a wall or a walking stick (Fig. 11.7). Walking sticks are often handed down from one family member to another, leaving the client with a stick of an inappropriate height. The stick may be too short causing them to stoop forward and off balance. The stick may be too high thereby not providing adequate support (refer to Chapter 7, Supported Living).

Activity 11.8 ■

Check with the physiotherapist that your client's walking aids are the correct height.
Check that the rubber ferrule has not worn through.

■ ■

Your client may require moral support while walking rather than physical support. If this is the case do not be tempted to link arms with them. If they become unsteady, you too may be pulled over. Simply stand at their

Fig. 11.7 Walking aids.

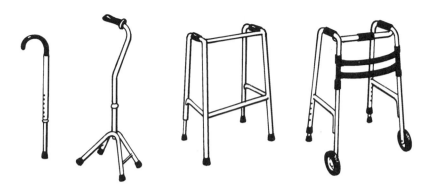

side and give verbal encouragement. If the client needs more support, the following methods can be used.

Carer assisting a client to walk

(1)   Stand on the weaker side of the client, stand to the side and slightly behind the client. If they have a weaker side then assist them on this side.
(2)   Place your arm closest to the client behind the client, around their waist and rest your palm on their hip.
(3)   Your other arm is used to support the client's hand closest to you, with the client's palm resting in yours (Fig. 11.8).

This position enables the client to lead the walk. The carer has control over the situation should the client feel faint or become unsteady.

Never attempt to catch or hold up a falling client as this could result in a serious injury for both the client and carer. The aim is to break the fall and let the client *slide* to the floor. This reduces the risk of injury to the client and prevents the risk of injury to the carer.

Controlling a fall

This technique should be demonstrated to you by an experienced practitioner.

If a client starts to sag while walking then:

(1)   Place your leg closest to the client behind them, keeping your knee slightly flexed.
(2)   Move your other leg further back to balance yourself.
(3)   As you do this move your arms under the client's axillae and bring the client back to rest on your thigh.
(4)   Lower your arms and allow the client to slide to the floor.

Fig. 11.8 Assisting client to walk.

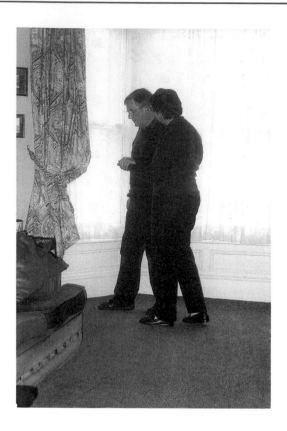

Able to maintain a sitting position

Knowing whether or not a client is able to maintain a sitting position unsupported, is of vital importance in relation to the method adopted for moving the client.

Moving a client from a lying to a sitting position

Many clients may be able to sit forward from the lying position by following simple instructions:

(1) Bend knees
(2) Roll on to side
(3) Push down with hands, bringing top part of body up

Where the client is unable to do this for themselves the following method can be used.

Note: the client must be able to control the movement of their head.

One carer and a towel are needed. If the client is heavier/bigger than the carer, then two are needed, one on either side.

(1)   Fold the towel in three lengthways.
(2)   Place it underneath the client's shoulders and around the upper part of their arms. Make sure it is not caught under the neck.
(3)   Work with the bed at the carer's knee level.
(4)   Facing the client put one knee on the bed at the level of the client's hip.
(5)   Hold both ends of the towel, close to the client's body.
(6)   Instruct the client to breath in on steady and out on sit.
(7)   On the command ready, steady, sit; the carer sits back on their heels using body weight to bring the client forward into the sitting position (Figs 11.9 and 11.10).

Fig. 11.9 Sitting a client forward
(a) starting position.

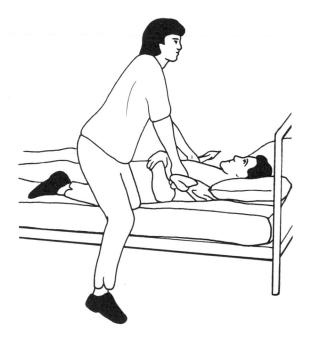

The bottom sheet on the bed can be used instead of a towel.

If the client is in an electronic bed, make the most of it to sit the client forward. Other equipment that may help the client bring themselves into a sitting position includes a monkey pole, or a rope ladder, attached to the foot of the bed. In the home the client may have handrails attached to the wall to assist with this activity. *Never* drag clients forward or up the bed by pulling on their arms.

Able to move up the bed

Before considering this, first think why clients slip down the bed? Two very common reasons are the traditional style back rest and the arrangement of pillows. The armchair arrangement is with one horizontal pillow, two diagonal and one horizontal. Does it sound familiar? Try it yourself. You

Fig. 11.10
(b) end position.

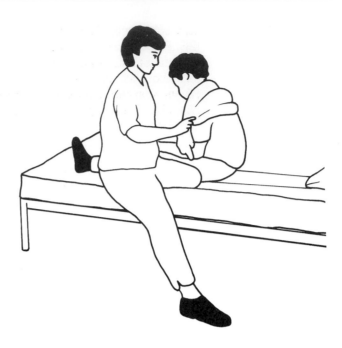

may find it restricts the expansion of your chest slightly, gives little support to the lower back and generally encourages you to slip down the bed, creating a shearing force between you and the bedclothes (refer to Chapter 10, Comfort and Rest). To reduce the chance of the client slipping down the bed, try positioning the pillows horizontally only and sit the client either upright or at a angle of 45°, not between the two.

Activity 11.9 ■

 Observe how the pillows have been arranged for the clients in your area.

■ ■

Note The sliding system referred to in the text is a loop of friction-free material specifically designed to aid in the moving of clients. This eliminates the need for carers to lift clients – a very dangerous practice for both parties.

Moving a client up the bed

The client should first be shown ways in which they can help themselves. By bending their knees slightly and rolling on to one side the client may be able to push themselves up the bed while on their side. This can be helped by the use of a friction-free sliding system placed at the side of the client, for them to roll on to. The client can then slide up the bed. The sliding system is removed as the client turns onto their back again.

Some clients may require a little more help. Equipment such as handblocks may help. By giving extra length to the arms the client is able to push themselves back up the bed.

An Australian slide is another alternative which enables the carers to slide the client up the bed (Fig. 11.11). This method is only suitable for clients who can maintain a sitting position. Two carers, a sliding system and a handling sling or a towel are required.

Fig. 11.11 Australian slide.

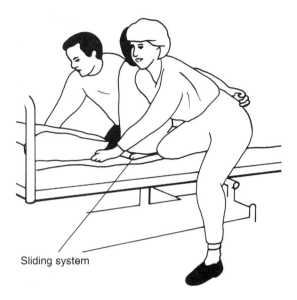

Sliding system

(1) Turn the client slightly from side to side to position the sliding system underneath the client's buttocks, ensuring excess material is at the back.

(2) Facing the head of the bed place, one knee on the bed parallel with the client's thigh and several inches beyond the client's back. This will depend on the height of the carer.

(3) The bed should be at a height that allows the leg on the floor to be flexed at the knee.

(4) The carer's arm nearest to the client is placed against their chest wall, just below the axilla.

(5) Place a handling sling beneath the client's thighs as close to the buttocks as possible. Hold the sling with the hand nearest to the client.

(6) The carer's free arm is put forward with the hand resting on the mattress. Keep this arm straight as it acts as a strut to ease stress on the carer's spine.

(7) At the start of the slide the carer should be sat back onto this foot.

(8) On the command ready, steady, slide the carer rises off her foot that is on the bed, keeping the handling sling sliding along the surface of the bed.

(9) The client is thus slid back in the bed.

(10) Turn the client slightly to either side to remove the sliding system.

Clients who are unable to maintain a sitting position without support, will need to be moved up the bed whilst lying flat or with the assistance of a hoist.

If the first method is to be used, a minimum of two carers will be required and a large sliding system. Work with the bed approximately at a level between the carer's hip and elbow.

(1)   Lay the client flat with one or two pillows under the head.
(2)   Wheel the bed out from the wall. Remove the bedhead.
(3)   Turn the client from side to side in order to position the sliding system under the bottom sheet. The sliding system needs to cover the area from just above the client's shoulder to just below the client's hips.
(4)   Two carers stand at the top of the bed with one leg forward of the other, body weight over the front leg, holding the bottom sheet at the level of the client's shoulders. On the command ready, steady, slide, the carers pull on the bottom sheet by transferring their body weight backwards. The client slides up the bed over the sliding system.
(5)   Turn the client to either side to remove the sliding system.
(6)   The client can then be sat forward using a towel or sheet. Pillows can be adjusted. A portable backrest may be needed to bridge the gap between the client and the backrest.
(7)   Rest the client back on the pillows.

Able to turn in bed

Can the client turn from side to side?

Some clients may be able to turn themselves to one side but not the other. If this is the case, always make use of what the client can do. Various pieces of equipment are available to help turn a client these include: turning slides, Rotaprone, and the Immoturn which can be used for turning clients following hip replacements.

Moving the client onto their side

This procedure is for activities such as washing, dressing or changing the sheets. The bed should be at a level between the carer's hip and elbow.

(1)   Turn the client away from you.
(2)   Turn the client's head to face direction of intended movement.
(3)   Bend the client's leg nearest to you, flop it over their other leg.
(4)   Place the client's arm nearest to you across their chest.
(5)   Position yourself with one hand on the client's hip and the other on their shoulder. Stand with one foot in front of the other and transfer your weight forwards pushing the client away from you onto their side. Ensure there is another carer on the opposite side of the bed or a cot side to prevent the client rolling out.

If turning the client towards you, place your hands on the client's hip and shoulder furthest from you. Transfer your body weight backwards and the client is rolled towards you onto their side (Fig. 11.12).

Fig. 11.12 Turning on to side.

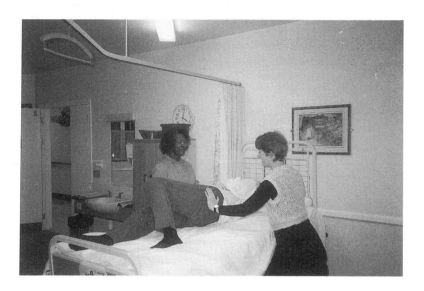

Moving the client for pressure relief

If the client is to be moved on to their side for pressure relief then a 30° tilt should be used. This position is usually very comfortable as the client is turned from soft tissue to soft tissue avoiding pressure on bony prominences. It can be used to relieve pressure when the client is lying flat or in a semi-reclined position. Work with the bed at the carer's hip and elbow level.

Two carers and a minimum of two pillows are required (not including those under the client's head).

(1) A carer stands either side of the bed
(2) Untuck the bottom sheet
(3) One carer holds the bottom sheet on the opposite side at the client's hip and shoulder level.
(4) The carer then pulls the client towards her to an angle of approximately 60°, using the sheet by transferring weight from front leg to back leg.
(5) The other carer places one pillow along the client's back and another along the length of the client's leg.
(6) The client then relaxes back against the pillows resulting in them being at an angle of 30°.

The client's final position should not exceed 60°. This is achieved by placing more of the pillow under the client.

Clients may require special beds or mattresses to help relieve pressure.

Standing from sitting

Points to remember:

- If a client is unable to weight bear and stand, NEVER attempt to stand them, as you will be supporting their entire weight.
- Consider the type of chair the client is in; a low, soft, easy chair is far more difficult to get out of than a high firm chair. The type of chair can make the difference between independence and dependence.
- A height-adjustable bed can be raised to a higher level, making it easier for the client to get out. Pillows and/or handblocks can be used either side of the client, acting as arm rests to aid the client into a standing position.
- A handling belt can be placed around the client's waist and used to assist them into a standing position.
- Standing and raising aids are also available. These are hoists that will bring the client into a standing position. The client must be able to weight bear through one or both legs.
- Chairs with seat raisers may also be appropriate for some clients.
- Never allow a client to place their hands around your neck when assisting them to move.

The client may just need simple guidance and encouragement to enable them to stand unaided as the following directions show.

(1) Wiggle forward in the chair.
(2) Position feet flat on the floor about hip distance apart, one foot in front of the other.
(3) Bring top part of body forward
(4) Place hands on arms of chair and push forward and up.

The following method can be used on clients whose assessment states they are able to weight bear and stand but have difficulty getting into the upright position. One or two carers may be needed. This will be determined by the initial assessment:

(1) The client needs to wiggle to the front of the chair.
(2) Place the client's feet apart with one foot slightly forward of the other.
(3) The carer stands at the side, facing the chair, with feet wide apart, knees flexed and one foot blocking the client's foot.
(4) The carer then places her shoulder nearest to the client against his chest wall, under the client's axilla and her arm around the client's waist.
(5) The client's arm can rest on the carer's back.
(6) The carer's free arm is placed on either the back or the arm of the chair, whichever is most comfortable.
(7) On the command ready, steady, stand, the carer will come into a standing position along with the client.

(8)   The client will be well supported.
(9)   If one carer is working on her own she should work on the client's less able side. The client will be required to push up on the arm rest with their more able arm (Fig. 11.13).

Fig. 11.13 Assisting client to stand (a) front view. (b) back view.

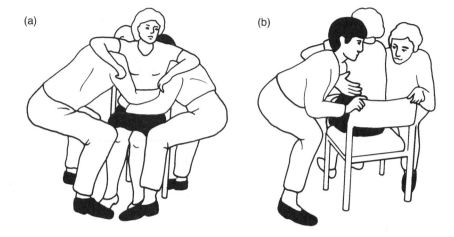

(a)

(b)

If a client is unable to weight bear and/or stand, they should be moved in a hoist or slid from one surface to another by using a transfer board and handling belt. This method could be used to move a client from bed to a chair/wheelchair from which the arm has been removed. NEVER manually lift a client.

Slipping forward in a chair

This is a similar situation to clients slipping down the bed, first consider why?

Perhaps the client doesn't find the chair comfortable. Maybe the seat is rubbing against their thighs. Perhaps pillows have been placed behind their back causing them to slip forward.

When seating a client, avoid placing pillows behind their back. Elevating the feet on a low footstool will not only prevent the seat from rubbing against the client's thighs but also help to maintain their upright position.

If the client has slipped forward consider whether they can move themselves back by using the following procedure:

(1)   Move their feet back (knees over toes).
(2)   Hold on to the arm rests and pull their top half forward.
(3)   The client then slides their bottom back in the chair.

Some clients may find it easier to stand up, take a step back and sit down again. A hoist could also be used.

Assisting the client to move back in the chair

If using this method ensure the chair is against a secure surface e.g. a wall, or get someone to hold the chair securely.

(1) Move client's feet back, knees over toes.
(2) Assist the client to fold their top half forward in the chair.
(3) Place a pillow lengthways against the client's knees and partly on their lap.
(4) Kneel on the floor in front of the client, sitting back on your heels.
(5) Place your hands on the pillow against their knees.
(6) Instruct the client to lean forward bringing their head towards the pillow.
(7) Rise off your heels pushing on the pillow against the client's knees and they will slide back in the chair.

Alternatively after (step 3)

(8) Stand in front of the client your toes pointing outwards, your knees against their knees cushioned by the pillow.
(9) Rest the client's hands on your waist.
(10) Place your hands under the client's axilla and gently fold them forward, at the same time push your knees against theirs to slide them back in the chair.

If a client has slipped too far forward in the chair it may be safer to slide them onto the floor, placing pillows on the floor before you do so. A hoist may then be used to raise the client from the floor.

Moving a client from the floor

Before attempting to move someone from the floor, first check to ensure they have not sustained any injury. Call a doctor or trained member of staff to do this. Once it has been decided it is safe for the client to be moved, make them comfortable. Either put a pillow beneath their head or sit them forward and place an upturned chair with pillows behind them as a temporary back rest. This will give the client time to recover and give you time to decide how you are going to move them, what equipment and help you require.

Once recovered the client may be able to get themselves up by using a chair and by following this procedure:

(1) The client bends their knees and rolls to one side.
(2) Pushes up on to all fours.
(3) A chair is then placed in front of them.
(4) The client then places their hands and forearms on the seat of the chair and moves slightly closer to the chair.
(5) Places their hands and forearms along the arm rests of the chair, then gently eases themselves up and round to sit on the chair.

If the client is unable to do this, then a hoist or booster cushion must be used if available to get them from the floor. If neither of these are available or the client is unable to go into a sitting position i.e. immediately following resuscitation after a cardiac arrest, then a minimum of six people, using a lifting sheet, strong counterpane or sheet are required to raise the client from the floor.

REMEMBER this method is a last resort:

(1) If possible move the bed and put the foot of the bed near the client's head.
(2) If possible remove the foot rest, apply the brakes and put the bed at almost its lowest level.
(3) Place the counterpane under the client by rolling them from side to side.
(4) Three carers work on either side of the client positioning themselves at head-shoulder, middle, knee-foot.
(5) The taller carers working at the head of the client the shorter at the foot.
(6) The carers kneel on one knee on the floor, one foot in front of the other, the front foot flat on the floor to maintain balance.
(7) Roll the counterpane close to the client and hold it with hands shoulder width apart, knuckles uppermost.
(8) The leader of the team gives the instructions ready, steady stand, and the team rises into a standing position.
(9) On the command ready, steady walk, the team walk towards the bed passing either side.
(10) Once the client is in position over the bed give the command ready, steady, lower and lower them onto the bed by the carers bending their knees.

Note: if you find it difficult to stand up from a kneeling position, do not participate in this technique as extra strain will be placed on your colleagues and the client would be at risk.

Hoists

The use of hoists should be planned into client care (Figs 11.14 and 11.5). There are a wide range of hoists available: mobile, fixed, overhead and portable. Carers should be given instruction on how to operate the hoists available to them and seen to be competent before using them on their clients. Clients can be apprehensive about the use of hoists and this may be increased if they see the carer is not sure of what they are doing.

Fig. 11.14 Sara hoist.

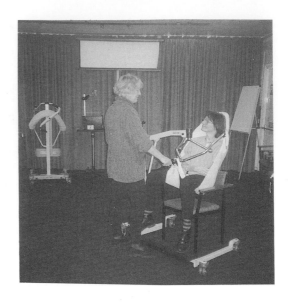

Fig. 11.15 Standing and raising aid.

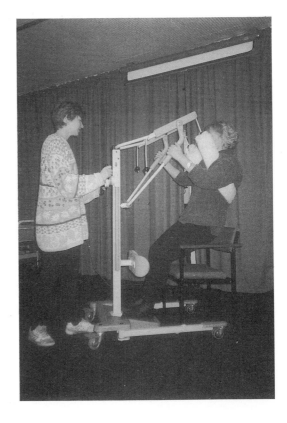

Activity 11.10 ■

What type of hoists are available in your area?
What is the maximum weight they can lift?
What type of slings are available?
When were the hoists last maintained?

■ ■

Clients can often be anxious about using a hoist due to a previous bad experience. Remember the purpose of a hoist is to transfer clients not transport them. Push the hoist by its handles or it may become unbalanced. Only raise the client high enough to clear the surface you are transferring from or to. Never leave a client unattended in a hoist. It may be helpful to show clients pictures of the hoist, or put yourself or a colleague in the hoist for the client to see. When showing a hoist to a client for the first time try to make it as small and inconspicuous as possible. If it is at its highest level with a sling draped across the front it can look very threatening.

Hoist Slings

Use the correct size sling for your client. This will depend on their weight and height. The type of sling used will also depend on the task to be performed and the clients' capabilities, e.g. toileting sling, bathing sling, amputee sling, stretcher sling. Take time to position slings correctly and ensure their are no wrinkles in the material. Always use the sling designed for the particular model of hoist you have.

Activity 11.11 ■

Ask a colleague to put you in the hoist. Consider what you liked/disliked about the experience. What would have made the experience better. This knowledge is often useful as you can explain how you felt and this may help to relieve some of your clients' anxieties.

■ ■

Bathing

A point to remember is that it is much easier to get into a bath than get out of one. Equipment available to assist includes:

- Bath seats
- Grab rails
- Booster seats
- Bath hoists

In some cases it may be necessary to change the bathroom into a walk/wheel-in shower room creating more space and easier access.

Toileting

We have already discussed ways in which the carer can assist the client to stand. However, in relation to the clients' mobility when using the toilet consider the following:

- Toileting slings
- Standing and raising hoists
- Grab rails/hand rails
- Raised ‚oilet seat
- Female/male urinals

Summary

I hope you have found this chapter useful. The most important thing to remember is to look after yourself so that you are fit to care for your clients. Legislation is there to protect you. Inform your manager if:

- Adequate assessments have not been performed on your clients.
- There is a change in a client's condition as this may effect their mobility.
- You have not received any formal training in manual and client handling.
- An adverse incident/accident occurs.

Finally, spend time planning and preparing for any manual handling activity both at work and at home.

References

Arfken, O.L., Lach, H.W., Birge, S.J. & Miller, J.P. (1994) Prevalence and correlates of fear of falling in elderly persons living in the community. *American Journal of Public Health*, April, **84**(4), 65–70.

Confederation of Health Service Employees (1992) *Back Breaking Work. A Survey on Back Injuries Among Health Care Workers*. COSHE, London.

Health and Safety Commission (1974) *Health and Safety at Work etc. Act 1974*. HMSO, London.

Health and Safety Commission (1992) *Manual Handling Operations 1992 – Regulations and Guidance*. HMSO, London.

Noble, L.J., Salcido, R., Walker, M.K., Atchinson, J. & Marshall, R. (1994) Improving functional mobility through exercise. *Rehabilitation Nursing Research*, Spring, **3**(1), 23–9.

Further reading

Ali, M. (1995) *Patient Handling Procedures for Nursing and Midwifery Staff*. UCL Hospitals NHS Trust.

Disabled Living Foundation. (1994) *Handling People Equipment, Advice and Information.* Disabled Living Foundation London.

Epiopoulos C. (1987) *Gerontological Nursing.* 2nd edn. J.B. Lipincott Company.

Isaacs B. (1992) *The Challenge of Geriatic Nursing.* Oxford Medical Publications.

McMahon, C. Harding, J. (1994) Chapter 5 in *Knowledge to Care*, Blackwell Science, Oxford.

Oliver, J. (1994) *Back Care.* Butterworth-Heinemann, Oxford.

Oliver, J. & Middleditch, A. (1991) *Functional Anatomy of the Spine.* Butterworth-Heinemann, Oxford.

Pheasant, S. (1991) *Ergonomics, Work and Health.* Macmillan Press Ltd, London.

Tarling, C. (1980) *Hoists and their Uses.* Heinemann, London.

Troup, J.D.G., Lloyd, P., Osbourne, C., Tarling, C. & Wright, B. (1992) *The Handling of Patients – Guide for Nurses*, 3rd edn. National Back Pain Association, Teddington.

Useful addresses

Disabled Living Foundation
380–384 Harrow Road
London W9 2HU

National Back Pain Association
16 Elmtree Road
Teddington
Middlesex TW11 8ST

Chapter 12
Recreation and Leisure Activities
Annette Drew

Overview

Recreation and leisure activities are not just a sing-a-long, bingo or games, but should be an integral part of the philosophy of care within a care environment. All clients whether they are in their own home or within an institutional setting need activities to shape their life. Many psychologists and nurse theorists include rest, work and play as essential activities of living. The important contribution of exercise to healthy living is not only recognized by medical circles but also promoted by the media.

■ The recognition of the older person as a skilled and interested adult with much to offer, encourages social interaction and personal development.
■ Careful planning of recreational and leisure programmes provide enjoyable exercise of both body and mind.
■ Carefully planned sessions encourage friendships, social interaction and creativity all contributing to a more fulfilled life-style.

Key words

Individuals, culture, activity, exercise, pleasure, skills, self-confidence, self-esteem, policy, leisure, communication, health, choice, dignity, creativity, role, memory, body image, social interaction, risk, assessment.

The importance of activities

Public perceptions of how older people spend their time still appear to be of passive and sedentary activity, preferably in isolated, private settings. It is also thought that people withdraw from active participation in public society and life once they retire.

Surveys show that older people perceive themselves as useful members of society, primarily involved with community activities, voluntary organizations, local politics and in helping to serve others (refer to Chapter 3, Relationships). Studies highlight the younger elderly as active in maintaining their networks of families and friends, in taking up new interests and maintaining existing hobbies. After retirement older people are reported to have more time to socialize with families and friends, and for such occupations as gardening, hobbies, walking and other recreational activities.

Few people reach later years without having created a physical and mental routine to their lives in a job or bringing up a family. People can experience stress and bereavement when these schedules and routines are disrupted or stopped, and this can lead to ill health and even premature death. Many studies have shown activity and exercise have healthy and positive effects on older people to counteract stress.

Activity 12.1 ■

Think about today, was there a time when you were doing and thinking about nothing?

■ ■

If there were gaps in your day, they were short and between events, you probably have set patterns to getting ready for work, doing house work, study, jobs around the house and other activities.

Older people often underestimate their capacity for exercise, thinking short sporadic episodes may be more advantageous. In many institutions, some carers often go further, believing exercise and activity are a luxury only available if time permits. If activities are provided, they are usually situated away from client areas and the few people attending are often the same each time. What is provided for those confined to their room or ward? Activity units away from the immediate client area have the advantage of specialist staff and club atmosphere. The disadvantage is care staff abdicate the responsibility for providing activities. Most activity units arrange sessions in the middle of the day, on weekdays, covering about 20 of the 168 hours in the week.

Exercise benefits the body mentally and physically.

The physical benefits provide

- Overall muscle toning and support
- Encourage better blood flow
- Decrease blood pressure and tension
- Decrease body fat percentage
- Improve heart muscle tone, respiration depth and rate therefore, gaseous exchange
- Digestion is improved by improved muscle tone, appetite control and bowel function
- Exercise induces natural sleep and is a factor in retarding progress of some degenerative diseases, e.g. rheumatoid arthritis

The mental benefits provide

- Improvement to mental ability
- Attention
- Memory
- Concentration and learning

Older people have the same mental abilities and skills as younger people, but they may take longer to acquire them. They learn in a different manner to younger people, learning more thoroughly and working longer. Severely disabled people do not lose these skills, but it may take a very long time for them to learn. Therefore, it is important to conform to prescribed action plans and to maintain learning or behaviour changing programmes for a long time.

Activities should be enjoyable, clients will only participate if it pleases them.

Activity 12.2 ■■■■■■■■■■■■■■■■■■■■■■■■■■■■■

List the activities you did yesterday.
Tick those giving you a lot of pleasure, cross off those you hated.
Do you have the larger list of neutral activities?
One way of improving your life is to plan an increase in those activities you enjoy the most.

■■■■■■■■■■■■■■■■■■■■■■■■■■■■■■■■■■■

Planning events for your clients is useless unless you know they will enjoy them. Assess clients to find out the things they enjoy doing. An activity programme should be organized around what the clients want, not the carer's idea of what they should do.

Activity 12.3 ■■■■■■■■■■■■■■■■■■■■■■■■■■■■■

Identify the organized events in your care area.
How much of the week is given to activities?
How many of these activities could your client choose to attend?

■■■■■■■■■■■■■■■■■■■■■■■■■■■■■■■■■■

Planning an activity programme

Activities should enable the older person to live a worthwhile, interesting and active life, while maintaining, as far as possible, their independence, self-esteem, determination, dignity and health.

Paramount to a successful activity programme is the philosophy of the care setting which includes the individuality of the client. Basic beliefs about the value of individuals and their contributions should be reflected in the organization of care. Beliefs and values acknowledge clients' right to dignity, privacy, self-determination, equality and choice. Valuing a person's own life experiences and personal worth foster a climate in which clients make choices about their life and activities. Staff should act as facilitators creating situations where clients achieve their goals. This may seem idealistic, but is fundamental to care planning aimed at improving the quality of life.

A successful activity programme needs the commitment of all carers. Staff and clients need to feel valued and feel that they have part to play. Some staff see activities as an easy option, failing to understand the amount of time necessary for the preparation and clearing away needed for a successful session. Success will not come easily, but it is a challenge to the clients and carers to make it interesting and enjoyable.

Check with managers the codes of practice, policies and procedures. All employees work within the rules of the work place, set to protect all concerned. Suggestions for activity should be planned within these limitations. Discover your own limitations and be aware of your skills. Check you understand what you are allowed to do, this may well be different from what you are capable of doing. Know your supervisors and make sure you understand agreed guidelines.

Activity 12.4 ■

List three ways of learning peoples' names.

■ ■

In many long stay establishments clients do not wear name badges or bracelets. If clients are coming from different areas or if they do not know each other, you may have some form of identification to begin with. The first activity could be to make name badges.

Be aware of the client's condition, this could be apparent from the assessment but if there are several different activity organizers, knowledge needs to be shared. If you are not sure about what clients can do, ask the person in charge. Drugs should not be handled by untrained staff, so if medication is due during a session or outing, consult the person in charge for the best way to handle the situation.

Assessment of the client should make their values and beliefs apparent. Clients with specific religious or cultural taboos should have this taken into consideration when planning activities. For example, Jehovah's Witnesses do not like to celebrate their own birthdays or anyone else's. They also do not celebrate Christmas or any other religious festivals throughout the year. Be sure to acknowledge and respect people's feelings.

Activity 12.5 ■

Which of your clients have special cultural needs?

■ ■

It is easy to become so engrossed in a project that we tend to forget others not so involved. Others may have a different focus for their attention. Put time aside to communicate with other staff and disciplines, to talk about your project and ideas to the team. Everybody has a busy schedule, so be aware of other staff. It is important to interest others in your project. Plan activities so they do not intrude into others' projects, environments or people's space. Ensure space or rooms are booked and communicate these intentions to others. Keep to time and tidy the area after use. Do not expect others to clear up after you, leave the space ready for the next group.

Activity 12.6 ■

How do you ensure the safety of equipment?

■ ■

Check all equipment and resources for safety. Remember older persons have delicate skin that tears and bruises easily. Be especially aware of sharp corners and implements, substances such as glue or paints, large pieces of equipment. Maintenance checks on all equipment should be made and recorded by the appropriate staff. Do not use equipment unless you are sure it is safe and that you know how to use it.

Commencing activities

Identify existing arrangements in other areas to prevent duplication. Physiotherapists hold exercise or music and movement sessions, the occupational therapists organize craft or games sessions, voluntary groups take sessions or clubs. Clients may not be currently attending for many reasons, discuss these with the person in charge before deciding if another group is needed.

Activity 12.7 ■

Using clients' assessments, make a list of activities the clients would like to be available. Which of these could you arrange? Which would you need help with? Have the clients got these skills?

■ ■

Many people underestimate their skills. Women often deny their cookery skills yet have successfully fed their families by reading and following recipes. Other departments may offer help.

Activity 12.8 ■

Consider who can contribute or help with an activity programme?

■ ■

Your list may include:

- Cashiers or cash holders
- Catering departments or kitchen
- Clergy, chaplain or priest, local church groups, youth clubs
- Clerical department or secretaries

■ Drivers and transport department
■ Laundry
■ Porters, receptionists
■ Social services

■ Switchboard or telephonists
■ Voluntary workers
■ Works department, maintenance

Make a directory of these people and their possible contribution and how to contact them. When producing the activity programme do not forget to add the names to your circulation list.

Activity 12.9 ■

 List the materials needed to start activities identified from your client assessments.

■ ■

■ Staff, friends and family, clients and relatives, suppliers all become sources from which to obtain materials.
■ A wanted poster in a prominent position will start your store, but do not forget to ask people personally (Fig. 12.1).
■ Circulars to all clients' relatives can sometimes help, also letters to suppliers can provide unused promotional material.
■ Discount coupons and promotions can be collected, local shops and suppliers often donate or offer discounts. Make your purchases from a school or handicraft wholesalers who are cheaper, but you may have

Fig. 12.1 A wanted poster.

WANTED
BY THE ACTIVITIES UNIT

Can you help with any of these items?

Atlases	Photography equipment
Board games	Anything about the World Wars
Books	Anything about the Royal Family
Cosmetics	Encyclopaedias
Craft books	Cookery and equipment
Flowercraft	Craft equipment
Foreign currency	Old cards, games, jigsaws
Gardening tools	Fabric and sewing material
Greeting cards	Gardening equipment
Knitting and crochet needles and wool	Old household appliances
Old mail order catalogues	Old clocks and watches
Old photographs	Pictures of sporting health
Travel books	Wool and silks
Crossword and quiz books	Wall paper
Ribbons and lace	Christmas paper
Records and tapes	Computer equipment

to buy in bulk. Think out the budget to make most of the money, crafts can be sold to buy more materials.

Budget

Consider the following:

- How much can be spent
- Who will fund the project
- Keep accurate accounts

Check-list

(1) Record all monies received from funding, donations, fundraising
(2) Issue receipts for donations and fundraising
(3) Keep a file for letters, e.g. thank you letters
(4) Keep a record of everything you spend and receipts
(5) If possible negotiate with the cashier to be involved for large items
(6) Only have a small petty cash account
(7) Buy large supplies monthly
(8) Think carefully about once only or annual purchases of equipment
(9) Keep the miscellaneous as small as possible

Activity 12.10   ■

Using the list of activities, consider equipment.
List the purchases you may need to buy

■ ■

Your list could include the following (Fig. 12.2):

- Scissors
- Paint brushes
- Artist easel
- Video recorder
- Slide projector
- Camera
- Books
- Enclyclopaedias
- Records

- Tapes
- Cookery equipment
- Gardening equipment
- Knitting needles
- Crochet hooks
- Basket making equipment
- Wood working tools
- Marquetry equipment

Hints on buying equipment

An increasing range of especially adapted equipment is available for many activities. For example, Help the Aged has a mail order catalogue. As most adapted equipment will be bought for specific individuals, make sure they can use it and will continue to do so for some time before buying. Equip-

Fig. 12.2 Some basic equipment.

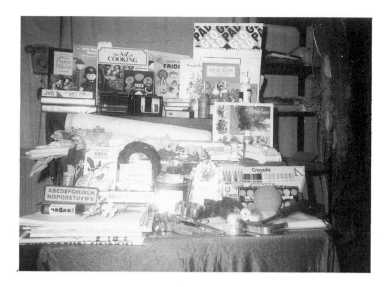

ment can be hired and it is worth investigating this approach before buying. Ordinary equipment can be adapted with ingenuity and thought. Wooden handles increase the diameter, foam and cord covering thin handles also increase the diameter and so the grip is made easier (refer to Chapter 7, Supported Living). Textured, colour-coded knobs and buttons help poor eyesight, and can be achieved with adhesive fabrics and papers.

Basic equipment

Basic supplies of *paper* paint, brushes, pencils and pens are essential. Local newspapers and printers sell end of rolls of newsprint.

Cosmetics can be donated from make-up parties. Muted colours are more popular but ask clients for their preference. Although a central storage is needed, a small case, tray or basket to keep items when attending a client is useful.

Food and *sundries* must be kept in airtight containers, some may have to be bought but many can be obtained from the kitchen, e.g. ice cream containers.

Cookery equipment, e.g. wooden rolling pins, shaped cutters, wire whisks, can be found at car boot or jumble sales.

Tape recorder and *camera*, are essential to record and remind people of the events at a later date.

Wipe clean floor mat games are a good buy, but find out what you could make yourself before buying. Waterproofed materials and fabrics and large checks are ideal for using for game boards. Large dice can be made from fabric covered boxes and if circular spots are too difficult, try continental squares. Large soft balls and counters are good buys and plastic picnic weights make very good counters.

Gardening tools should be lightweight with broad handles. A raised garden area is best for wheelchair bound clients (Fig. 12.3). Long handled tools are available for disabled people. Only buy what you currently need and find out if you need to make other purchases as you go along.

Fig. 12.3 Using a raised garden.

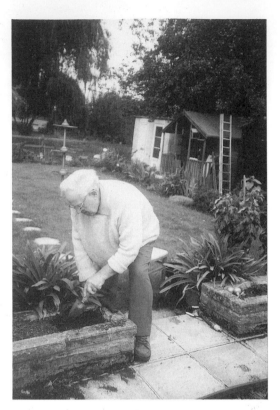

Other activities

Flower arranging can be undertaken indoors in all weathers and made purposeful by inviting clients to take responsibility for the selection and arranging flowers for the dining room table or chapel. Potted plants and bulbs are simple to plant and a pleasure to watch growing.

Exercise programmes set to music and prerecorded are available. Choose music to suit individual taste and in keeping with the client group. Percussion instruments give an added interest to sessions.

Cards, dominoes, draughts and chess are popular pastimes. Games based on popular television programmes are available, but select those with less detail to prevent tiring and confusing clients with poor eyesight.

Assessing a client

Assessing clients before arranging an activities programme or buying equipment is essential. This is undertaken by a qualified person with the carer's help. Clients have very different ideas from carers, relatives and friends about what they would like to do. Short client profiles can be updated as you get to know the client better. Information collected about clients should be specific to activity programmes. Do not duplicate information already in clients' notes and care plans. Collecting information about clients can invade privacy so should be kept to the minimum for the purpose.

Activity 12.11 ■

List the questions you would like to ask a client.
Which are the three most important, do they give you enough information to plan an activity?

■ ■

Use all your communication skills to listen to the client. Choose a quiet, unhurried time and place with comfortable chairs and listen to the client. Many older, infirm or disabled people think carers know best, but not so in this case. Only the client knows their interests, what they have enjoyed in the past, would like to try, or never had a chance of doing. Clients with communication difficulties need extra time spent with them. Ask permission of the client, for information to be obtained from family and friends (refer to Chapter 2, Communications).

Method of assessment

- Obtain permission to collect information before you start.
- Ask client's preferred mode of address.
- Explain purpose of assessment and discuss issues of confidentiality.
- Information is usually collected on a chart, but explore other methods, especially when caring for clients who have difficulty communicating.
- Observe and record how clients enjoy events, watch their reactions to food and drinks, how long they can sit comfortably or concentrate on one activity.
- Consider the distance from the television, how close do they need to be in order to see and hear; is the radio at the correct volume?
- Encourage clients to be involved in assessment, show them the programme and encourage participation; ask them to perform simple small tasks to demonstrate ability.
- When information is gathered and collated, return to the client to check accuracy.

People and circumstances change, assessment undertaken several months previously may not be currently accurate as clients' conditions change. People become bored or disinterested in activities they are involved with, so it is important to reassess regularly.

In some organizations tests, check lists and score charts may be used to help assess physical or mental ability or a combination of both (Fig. 12.4).

Fig. 12.4 Activities assessment chart.

Assessment sheet

Name: Likes to be called:

Room: Spends the day:

ABILITIES/HEALTH

Physical:

Mental:

Sight:

Hearing:

Taste:

EDUCATION/SCHOOLING

Would like to learn:

Library books:

ACTIVITIES

Currently doing:

None in the past:

Would like to do:

RELATIVES AND FRIENDS

Normally visit:

Would help with:

Would accompany on outings:

Could bring a car:

Starting a group

Little is gained from organizing activities without knowing clients' preferences. Decisions about activities should arise from discussion about future events. Ideas generated should be discussed further with clients checking their needs before spending time planning. Goals should be clear and organizers confident they can undertake the task. Group work is very demanding and carers need time to be supportive of each other, to unwind, review their feelings and listen to each other's needs.

Planning the session

Planning and preparing for the session takes twice as long as the session itself.

Where sessions are held will be dictated by the type of session. Planting spring bulbs in the lounge where the compost could damage the carpet may be inappropriate!

When planning a session, the following considerations need to be discussed:

- Hard or soft surfaces, washable floors
- Equipment, size of group
- Types of chairs and tables
- Lighting and heating
- Mix of group, amount of supervision, number of helpers required

Some special units have different areas for types of activities or adaptable areas. It is preferable to split the group and hold two sessions than to have too large a group. The mix of people is important, so that they can work together. There may be some occasions, when clients of differing ability can be managed together, those needing less supervision can be left to get on with a task while attention can be focused on more dependent clients.

Clients of similar ability form better groups, each carer can help one or two highly dependent clients needing a lot of supervision, or two or four medium dependent clients. This is only a rough guide, since this will vary according to the type of activity session, the client's personality and ability.

Heavily dependent clients may be those who have been living alone or in an establishment without an activity programme. Choose people carefully for each group, making an activity programme a success is achieved by keeping within the abilities of individuals. Choose activities that clients want to attend, use the information from their assessment profile. Make the first tasks challenging but pleasurable and when tasks are completed ensure they have something to take home or can keep.

Content of session

When choosing clients for a group, age is not so important as ability. However, age is very important when deciding the content of the session. Music, pictures or themes focusing on the client's prime years, highlight the difference between the experience and culture of the 1940s and the 1960s. A 20 year gap in younger people tends to become less important in the eyes of carers as people get older, but this is not so with the clients.

Within periods of time individual experiences were very different. Not everyone was involved with the flower power or hippie cults of the 1960s or had good or bad times during the war. People of different backgrounds knew very different worlds. The media was less invasive 50 years ago and there was less social mobility, so clients may have little knowledge of the kind of life of people led at the other end of their own town.

Remember, all clients have traditional and religious backgrounds, and for some this is very strong. They may or may not wish to share this aspect of their lives but all carers must respect the individuality of each client. Be aware of special days both for the individual and within cultural calendars.

For the age group we are caring for the genders did not mix as they do today, many older people find it difficult to mix with the opposite sex. Men and women had defined roles in life, and social traditions and taboos have to be observed. It is difficult for some older people to engage in mixed activities, and for spinsters and bachelors this may be even more difficult. Many older people find the fashion of mixed wards embarrassing and difficult to understand. When starting groups, attend to the social graces of introduction, if you are not sure of the etiquette, ask your clients – they know. This will give the client control and may help them to accept mixed social activities.

When planning groups, it is important to obtain the correct mix of clients. A large group with plenty of helpers enables a broader range of skills, ability and concentration span to be managed. Small groups which concentrate on specific tasks require members to be of similar ability.

Clients not attending activities

People refusing to attend activities still need to be asked and be able to refuse. Saying no is as much of a choice as saying yes. Note the reasons they give. Check these reasons with the client at a later date so it is not seen as pressuring the client.

Discuss the reasons for not participating. Is it:

- Lack of interesting activities
- Difficulty in meeting others
- Having disabilities which embarrass them

Consider their answers, would a one to one session suit them better?

Meeting the needs of the disabled client

More disabled clients may need special activities to be arranged in their immediate environment with increased carer support. Sessions need to be:

- Short
- Well organized
- Suitable level of manual dexterity
- Include all senses, including taste, smell, sight, hearing and touch. Sensual stimulation is especially important for those clients with communication difficulties
- One to one sessions within a group session. This quality time, however

short, is worth a great deal more than group time and it is surprising how quickly people will respond.

■ Do not forget those who appear not to communicate can still hear, taste, smell, touch and see.

Suitable activities for disabled clients

All types of activities can be adapted to suit most environments. For instance, theme days such as a French day. This could include French music, food, coffee, clothes; how about decorating the area with French flags, onion strings, posters, or dressing up in sailor shirts and berets? It does not have to be complicated, but those attending can join in as they wish while the theme goes on around them.

Reminiscence therapy

Reminiscence therapy requires trained therapists, but the principles and use of reminiscence can be incorporated into other groups and sessions.
    Reminiscence is:

■ A healthy and therapeutic review of life events
■ Remembering one's life events
■ Recounting experiences
■ Reflecting on life history

    Psychologists believe that everyone indulges in life in reminiscences and life history narration. Children recall and reflect upon life events as part of learning. In later life the relationship between past and the future changes, the past becomes greater than the future and takes on an added significance. Erikson's stages of development in man identifies the seventh stage of adult life as having a generative function and the eighth as that of reviewing with pride or despair the accomplishments of life. Oral and written histories may be part of the generation of legacies to be handed on to the next generation. Sharing one's own life history as one approaches the end of life helps in the process of review and coming to terms with one's contribution's to family, society and the world. An essential feature of social life is the sharing of experiences. Oral and written histories keep a person alive in the minds of others. Everyone has a life story and while being famous through the media is not for all, many people achieve fame within their own family circle.

Case study 1

John was 84 years of age when he undertook to writing his own personal account of his life. This included his education, marriage, family and building up a small business. One of his daughters-in-law typed it up. It was copied, bound and distributed to John's four children. On reflection

John found it a very therapeutic exercise to give this account of his life and felt satisfied, while his family had a lasting memento of their father's life and work.

- Autobiographies
- Tape recorded memories
- Scrapbook life histories
- Photographs

All these are important to help people remember and give value to their lives. Such records are helpful for those clients who find it difficult to remember their lives. Although each person has an individual personal history, they were also part of a generation so have a collective history. Each person will react differently to events of their age. One person may feel important for their contribution to the war while another may only have memories of pain, hurt and deprivation.

The years of youthful idealism, of our prime, of building a career and family are most deeply imprinted in our minds. They tend to be remembered with a rosy glow, remembering the best and glossing over the bad parts. They were the years of building one's identity and finding meaning and direction to life. These memories are highly influenced by the fashions and natural events and trends of the time. It is important to remember that the older people, who we as carers put together in groups for care or recreational purposes, all have very different memories from different eras. Five to ten years can make a lot of difference when recalling music, fashions, status and world events. As the pace of change increases these differences will become more pronounced.

Personal possessions

These are highly charged with memories and meaning that should be valued and treasured, providing a focus for helping clients to remember. Encourage clients to tell their family and friends what they would like to do with these objects when they die.

Case study 2

Following Winnie's death, her family were looking through Winnie's jewellery box and found that most items had been labelled with the names of various people within the family. This former action of Winnie not only made it easier to share her treasured belongings, it also meant they were disposed of as she had wished and all the family had a valued memento of Winnie.

It is important to older people to think about their legacies whatever they are. A verbal history of objects is of great worth and equally important to the owner.

Reminiscence groups

Reminiscence groups use memories in a therapeutic manner by helping to make sense of their lives, sort out old discrepancies and to come to terms with old events. Reminiscence can trigger good and bad memories so the group leader must be prepared to deal with pleasure and pain. Tears can often be therapeutic so should be allowed appropriately, a counsellor should be used if the carer does not have these skills. Topics should be universal to enable all the group to participate and contribute.

The group should be of similar people with enough carers to deal with distressed clients should this occur. Often the group will decide on a theme, using articles to trigger memories. The group leader ensures all clients have a space to talk. The group should meet regularly to promote memory and provide a safe group in which clients recall their lives.

Items to stimulate a group or one to one session.

- Newspaper headlines
- Old post cards
- Clients' own possessions

Themes

Larger, or more prolonged sessions can use themes to help stimulate memories and encourage social skills and all the senses.

- Themes can be a single session or linked events over a period of time.
- Choose a theme that most clients can relate to and that has been suggested by the group.
- Collect together objects that will stimulate all the senses.
- Use items that the clients bring to the group, this helps the client to feel valued and involved.
- Keep concentration span within the ability of the group, two small sessions are better than one long one.
- Prepare well in advance, collect materials and file topics. Never throw away a magazine until you have saved any relevant pictures, colours, ideas you can use at a later date.
- Items for touch may include fabrics, fur, feather, shells, silk, hard and soft, rough and smooth.
- 'Smellies' can include bottles of perfume, lavender water, spices, peppermints, mothballs.
- Record sounds on tape, steam engines, motor bikes, bird song, children playing for example.

Many local museums have themes and articles you can borrow, a deposit against loss or damage may be required (Figs 12.5 and 12.6).

Activity 12.12 ■

Choose a theme and collect materials for use in a session.

■ ■

Fig. 12.5 Some ideas for themes.

Themes for Activity Sessions

Art	Autumn
Anniversaries	Animals
Birds	Books and stories
Childhood	Christmas
Countryside	Current affairs
Colour	Craft and hobbies
Easter	Entertainments
Fashion	Famous people
Famous buildings	Films
Foreign travel	Fund raising
Garden	Good grooming
Halloween	Housework
Homes	History
Holidays	Healthy living
Indoor games	Industry
Ladies' day	Mothers' Day
Money	Music
Newspapers	New Year
Old crafts	Other cultures
Old boys' day	Other countries
Pets	Party times
Poetry	Pub signs
Royalty	Religion
Seaside	Sports
School days	Spring
Summer	Silent movies
Transport	Television
Weather	Winter
World events	World wars
Weddings	Wireless and radio

Collect articles to stimulate all the senses, taste, touch, smell, hearing and sight. Try to get some old items, ask clients relatives and friends for help. Approach the local library or museum.

Themes can link many activities and sessions together. An example could be fruit picking:

- Get or make a local map
- Take clients to 'pick their own fruit'. Many may not be familiar with this.
- Take photographs
- Show photographs to others and tell them of the trip
- Make jams or pies
- Have a tea dance to share them
- Plan another trip

Fig. 12.6 Materials for a wedding theme.

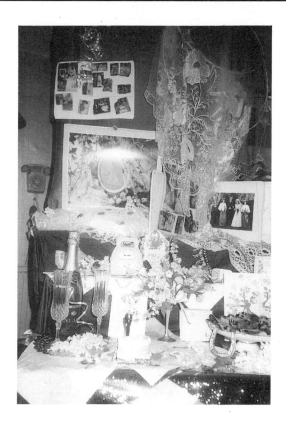

Activity 12.13 ■

 List the different activities could be included in this theme.

■ ■

Your list could include:

- Exercises
- Practice movements
- Practice of memory and thinking
- Social skills
- Conversation

All activities should be pleasurable and enjoyable (Fig 12.7).

Activities suitable for less skilled or able clients

Alternative therapy

This encourages a sense of well-being and relaxation and creates a feeling of inner peace. They can also improve hand and eye co-ordination and exercise the upper body.

Fig. 12.7 A week of activities.

ACTIVITIES PROGRAMME

Day	Morning session	Afternoon	Evening
Monday	Music and movement *dr* Hairdresser	Residents committee *lo* Post Office trip	Bingo *dr* Card making *dr*
Tuesday	Gardening club *con* Aromathrapy *lo*	Classical music *lo* Craft club *dr*	Video club *dr*
Wednesday party	Wheelchair aerobics *dr*	Shopping trip	Card Whist drive *dr*
Thursday concert	Relaxation classes *lo*	Reminiscence group *lo*	Carol practice *dr*
Friday	Music and movement *dr*	Pottery class *con*	Pub Quiz night *lo*
Saturday	Relatives and ramblers picnic lunch at Red Lion Cookery *dr*		Sing along *lo*
Sunday	Church at St Johns Boot fair *con* and car park.		Songs of Praise

dr – dining room   *lo* – lounge   *con* – conservatory

Therapies include:

- Aromatherapy
- Massage
- Relaxation therapies
- Crystal therapies
- Reflexology

Before trying any of these therapies consult the person in charge and trained therapists and ensure you comply with any local policies. The use of smell can be therapeutic and pleasing. Simple use of oils as relaxation aids can induce sleep (refer to Chapter 10, Sleep and Rest). Careful use of oils in burners, the bath and under pillows requires little in the way of equipment, but should be supervised by trained therapists. Some oils are poisonous so careful storage is essential. Use tapes of voice and poetry or music to create a relaxing atmosphere, breathing exercises, reminiscence and fantasy to create relaxation.

Art and drawing

This gives people a sense of achievement, creates beauty and enhances the environment. It encourages fine hand movements, hand and eye co-ordination.

- Art Painting
- Drawing
- Sketching
- Collage
- Marbling

- Stencilling
- Stamp art
- Visit to art galleries
- Art appreciation sessions

For people with little artistic skill, have poor co-ordination or poor fine movement, they try some of the following and obtain excellent results.

- Group picture, directly drawing or painting onto a background, colouring in already prepared outlines
- Stencils to give outlines to designs and for use on both paper and fabrics
- Stamp art using pre-made rubber stamps to give an outline that can be coloured or printed directly onto papers and fabrics.
- Colouring in shapes to add to a group picture
- Marbling uses special paints and dyes floated on a medium to transfer the design from the bath to paper or fabrics and can be used for all levels of skill.

Basket work

This can create beautiful and useful items giving a sense of achievement and improves finger and hand strength and dexterity. Basket work includes basket weaving, decorating, cane seats for stools and chairs.

Baskets made with a mixture of fabrics, ribbons and raffia give an alternative for less strong fingers. Decorate baskets with painting or stencils. Stiff type bows and biscuit porcelain flowers are also very fashionable decorations.

Beauty

This encourages good grooming, self-awareness and improves morale, (refer to Chapter 10, Hygiene). Beauty treatments include hair dressing, manicures, pedicures, facials.

Check with your organization's policy on nail cutting, nearly everyone enjoys the attention that a manicure can give. Should nail varnish be used, ensure it is a colour of the client's choice.

Calligraphy

Calligraphy maintains and develops old skills and creates beautiful items. These include making cards, illuminated scripts, decorating paper crafts.

Calligraphy pens are now made like felt tip pens making them easier to use. Many older people were taught good hand writing e.g. copperplate and this will remind them of previous skills.

Cookery

This maintains and values old skills, encourages creativity and memory. It also exercises the arm, shoulder and upper body. Cookery ideas include.

- Deciding on the recipe
- Making a shopping list
- Shopping or fruit picking
- Cooking and making occasions of the eating, e.g. tea party, tea dance

For people unable to manage the whole process, cutting out biscuits or cakes from ready-made mixtures can be just as much fun.

Current affairs

This promotes awareness of national and local events, encourages memory and brain activity, encourages participation and sharing of ideas and opinions. It also promotes respect for other people's personal beliefs and ideas. Ideas for sessions on the topic include:

- Newspaper reading
- Using headlines as debate or quiz topics
- Visit to local museums, libraries or historical places
- Video shows of events
- Making a celebration of anniversaries of national events

Start by arranging small groups as some people find it difficult to speak in large ones. Games based on newspaper cuttings, such as matching headlines, talking about topics, listing things about events will encourage people to contribute; or just sit with the clients over coffee and read the headlines to them and discuss the events.

Dancing

This encourages physical activity, social skills and interaction. Suggestions include:

- Country dancing
- Barn dances, tea dances
- Talking about old dances
- Demonstration dances

Simple dance steps set to music as part of an exercise programme can stimulate client interest. Arrange tea dancing, watch videos of different types of dancing.

Decoupage

This decoration of different surfaces with paper cut-outs encourages a sense of creativity. Decoupage includes decorating cards, household objects and furniture.

Pictures can be cut out from magazines, cards or bought from specialist producers. Recycling trays, waste paper baskets and other small objects keeps costs low. Start with cards, calendars and small projects. Those who find it difficult to cut out can still paste and varnish.

Fabric painting

This encourages creativity and improves hand-eye co-ordination and manual dexterity. Cotton, silk, synthetics can all be painted.

Garments such as scarves and T-shirts are cheap and easy to start with. Fabric paints should be correct for the type of fabric. Domestic irons can now be used for stabilizing the paints, check them when buying. Fabric paints come in pen and crayon styles that are easier to hold. For small projects needlework frames can be used to hold the fabric.

Flowercrafts

These maintain and value old skills, they also encourage creativity. The activity exercises arms and upper body. Flowercrafts include:

- pressed flowers
- dried flowers
- dried seeds heads
- cards

- pictures
- flower displays
- collage
- pot pouri

Drying petals and flowerheads for pot pourri are simple, but satisfying tasks. Bought dried flowers can be used to make cards, pictures and calendars, or decorate household objects (Fig. 12.8). Telephone books are a cheap way to start flower pressing.

Do not forget to ask permission before cutting flowers, and remember some plants are poisonous.

Fundraising

This encourages a sense of self-esteem, self-worth and achievement. Contributing to the well-being of others, group effort and social skills. Fundraising ideas include:

- Raffles
- Jumble sales
- Sales of work
- Craft sales
- Car boot sales

- Sponsored events
- Concerts
- Pub quizzes
- Competitions

Check with managers concerning any policies on fundraising. Commence with small easy-to-manage events such as raffles. Use the skills of the clients, many will have experience in this field. Decide before you start

Fig. 12.8 Flowercraft
materials.

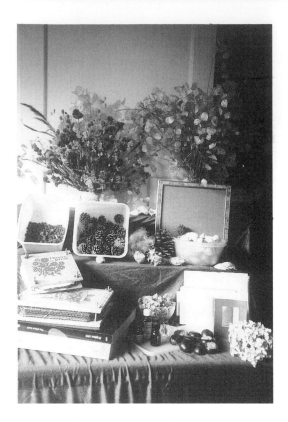

where the money will be donated and make this clear to the participants
and donors. Do not forget to publish the results and to thank donators.

Gardening

Gardening maintains and values old skills, gives a sense of achievement
and clients can enjoy the fruits of their labours. Gardening exercises the
hands and upper body. Activities include:

- Indoor and outdoor gardening
- Pot plants
- Bulbs
- Tomatoes in 'grow bags'
- Flower arranging

Pot plants, tubs and boxes are useful, if no raised garden is available.
Start with easy projects such as planting bulbs or tomato shoots, so participants can enjoy the results. Some people may like to help the gardener,
if there is one, or be responsible for part of the garden.

Housecraft

This maintains a sense of worth, giving a sense of achievement. It exercises
the whole body.

Housecraft activities include:

- Dusting
- Setting tables
- Keeping own room tidy

- Answering the front door bell
- Tidying lounge areas
- Helping with teas

Many clients miss the normal routine of keeping house. Ensure others do not follow round after the clients as this is very demoralizing. Carers often underestimate clients' ability to undertake household tasks.

Jewellery

This gives a sense of achievement, heightens awareness for grooming, and appreciation of beautiful things. This activity helps fine hand movements. The activity can include:

- Appreciation of gems
- Making jewellery
- Cleaning jewellery

- Talks on gems
- Demonstrations

Knitting and crochet

Knitting and crochet maintain and value old skills and encourage memory and thinking skills. The activity help fine hand movements. Activities include:

- Making garments
- Toys
- Squares for blankets

Making items for personal use, fundraising or use within the organization gives a sense of achievement. Many clients have skills, but may need to use larger needles, try 'broomstick' knitting. People can be taught knitting and crochet with one mobile hand and using the disabled hand to steady the work.

Ladies' circle

This encourages memory and thinking skills, social skills and organizational skills and promotes awareness of current affairs. Activities can include speakers on different topics and visits to local groups.

Networking with existing community groups maintains links with the local community. Arrange speakers to visit the clients, or develop a programme. Women's Institute and Towns Women's Guilds will help start groups.

Memory groups

These encourage memory, thinking and social skills. Activities include:

- Kim's game
- Alphabet games
- Feely bag
- Word games
- Quizzes

Making games can also be part of the activity programme, paper plates make bases to put pictures on for matching or pairing games. Large items to be played on the floor with a pointing stick, increase exercise and body movements. Memory can be improved with use, so include clients with memory loss, but adapt games to keep within their concentration span.

Model making

This gives a sense of achievement and maintains and values old skills. It is a good activity to increase hand and finger movements. Suggestions include:

- Model kits
- Cardboard models
- Dolls houses
- Aeroplanes
- Talks from model makers or groups
- Demonstrations

Kits are good to start with, but look for simple models with larger pieces. Model-making groups will give advice. Talks from model makers are interesting and they also display their work. You will find that clients already have many skills that can be adapted to model making.

Music

Music encourages memory and thinking skills. It also encourages appreciation of beauty, relaxation and enjoyment. Activities can include:

- Music and movement
- Music appreciation
- Sing-a-longs
- Concerts
- Making music

Music and movement tapes can be bought with instructions for specific groups. Later, you can compile your own selections, but make sure the music is compatible with the clients. Know your clients' tastes and put together taped concerts. Many local music groups will come and give concerts. Visit a concert at local venues.

Needlecraft

This maintains and values old skills and gives a sense if achievement. The activity is good for hand and fine finger movements. Needlecraft includes:

- Embroidery
- Tapestry
- Plastic canvas
- Lace making

- Punch crafts
- Beading
- Rug making

Crafts can be adapted for clients with limited movements. Plastic canvas can be used instead of normal canvas and made into useful household objects. Being stiff it can be fastened to a table or frame for working. Table and floor frames for holding the fabric are helpful for people who find it difficult to hold the work (Fig. 12.9). Rug canvas can be attached to frames and although it needs stronger fingers, it is large to see. Punch craft uses tools with handles that can be enlarged for easier manipulation. Photo-copying can enlarge patterns.

Fig. 12.9 Tapestry on a floor frame.

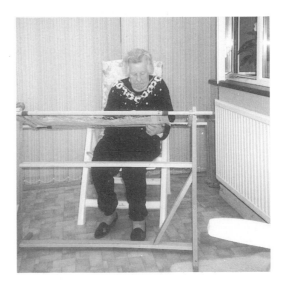

Outings

Outings encourage memory and thinking and social skills and awareness of community. Suggestions include:

- Local shopping
- Visits to museums and galleries
- Parks and picnics
- Schools and colleges

- Libraries
- Visits to farms and local events
- Shows
- The seaside

Start with local shopping trips, pub lunches, local parks with small numbers of clients. Many older people have never visited larger super-markets with café and toilet facilities. Contact the manager and find out quieter times, they are usually very helpful in extending extra help.

Schools and colleges put on exhibitions and events, your clients could reciprocate with oral history sessions. Theatres and conference centres have good facilities for disabled people and wheelchair access. Contact the manager to discuss outings and reduced rates.

Paper craft

This gives a sense of achievement, encourages memory and thinking skills. Ideas include:

- Cards
- Calendars
- Pictures

- Decoupage
- Origami

Recycling old cards into new cards, calendars and pictures can be satisfying and requires few skills. Victorian skills of decorating household objects with picture scraps has come back into fashion and can provide an interesting pastime. Using magazine pictures reduces costs while skills are learned.

Pets

Pets promote a sense of caring, tactile warmth and relaxation (Fig. 12.10) Ideas include:

- 'Pat a dog'
- Pets corner
- House pets

Many older people have to give up their pets when they enter residential care and suffer severe bereavement. House or visiting pets can provide tactile experience and a chance to care for a pet. Research shows that stroking animals can reduce stress and tension.

Fig. 12.10 Pets induce relaxation.

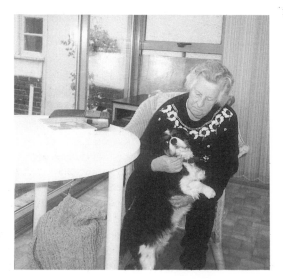

Pottery

This activity promotes creativity and gives a sense of achievement. It is a good form of hand and arm exercise. Suggestions include:

- Clay
- Newclay
- Plasticine
- Salt dough
- Modelling

- Ceramics
- Painting plates
- Visits to local potteries and china exhibitions

Using any of the materials is good therapy for hand and fingers. Newclay can be baked in a domestic oven, check when buying. Ceramics can be bought ready made for painting and make good fundraising items. Painting ordinary domestic crockery is very satisfying and relatively inexpensive.

Pre-discharge group

This gives confidence for those clients in residential care to return to the community and keeps links with the community. Activities include:

- Discussion groups
- Outings to shops

- Orientation outings
- Visits home and to locality

Discussion groups where anxieties above returning home can be aired will help clients bridge the gap between sheltered residential care and taking up responsibilities at home. Visits home to familiarize clients with home living will help to build confidence. Outings to local facilities will help clients to readjust.

Reality orientation

This maintains and improves memory and orientates clients to present day events and situations. Activities include reality orientation groups, including reality orientation ideas within other groups. Refer to previous discussion of this topic in Chapter 2, Communications.

Social skills

Social skills promote awareness, communication and assertiveness. This activity can take place either in role play or group discussion.

A long mirror is essential as it encourages clients to see themselves when practising their behaviour skills. Set up situations that clients can practice, e.g. taking goods back to a store or going to the post office. Start with ordinary situations in which clients need to achieve social skills for independent living. Visits to shops and pubs help clients to observe other people in everyday situations. Use verbal and non-verbal communication games, such as making up a group story or consequence games. Another activity is dancing which allows people to experience touch.

Sport

This encourages memory and thinking skills, provides exercise and movement and develops team and group skills. Suggestions include:

- visits to sporting events
- watching sport on television or video
- sponsored sporting events
- sports club
- support a local team

Make sport on television a purposeful occasion, prepare for it, watch in groups and have a discussion afterwards with refreshments. Create a sports club or league for tiddlywinks championships, indoor bowls or table tennis tournaments, sponsored skittles matches, darts, dominoes, or table games. Create supporters clubs for local teams, organize fundraising, outings to matches. Make an occasion of national events, hold sweeps, encourage groups to support different teams, hold discussion groups on sport, organize visits by local players or teams.

Video club

This can provide enjoyment, develop choice, and teaches clients to work with others. It also encourages memory, tolerance and patience. The activity includes borrowing videos from a local shop and going to the local cinema.

Start with borrowing from local video shops or libraries, then get clients to choose the next video. Gradually build up your own library by recording old films.

Voluntary work

This encourages memory and thinking skills and offers the opportunity to give to others. Suggestions include:

- Serving tea at local occasions
- Helping in shops or on stalls
- Making items for sale

Many people have been volunteers and may wish to continue, liaise with managers of local charities for suitable duties the client can comfortably carry out. Fundraising may take the place of an active involvement, always ensure clients attend some the events.

Keeping records

Keeping records is an essential part of every carer's day. It helps to analyse and reflect on activities undertaken. Make notes on each activity:

- Where and when it was held
- Who attended
- Client's interaction, who they spoke to, spontaneous conversation, interests in common

- Levels and span of concentration
- Note improvements for future activities
- Make reminders for future activities

Ideally, information should be kept in the client's notes or care plans. However, if this is neither possible nor convenient, then notes should be kept in the activity unit (Figs 12.11 and 12.12).
You can use:

- Charts
- A diary

- A log type record
- Kardex

Activity 12.14 ■

List the information you would keep about a client to help you plan for future events.

■ ■

Your list could include:

Record what the client enjoyed:

- Type of activity
- Parts of the activity most enjoyed
- Managed most easily
- Understood
- Remembered

How well did the client cope:

- With other clients
- Interaction between client and carers
- Social skills

Records show progress of groups and individuals within that event, which helps future planning. Ensure that records are available for inter-departmental liaison, as it saves duplication.

Relatives and friends need to know the progress of clients. A photograph collection can help with communication, especially if the client suffers from communication difficulties, as this will help to focus the conversation.

For clients with memory problem, a diary recording client activities helps relatives to keep in touch. Encourage relatives to contribute, so that when clients forget an event they can be reminded.

Fig. 12.11 Client's
activity record.

CLIENT'S RECORD OF ACTIVITY

Client . . . .   **Date:** . . . .

Activity

Eagerness to attend:
0   Refused to come
1   Needed persuasion
2   Needed reminding
3   Came unprompted

Memory span:
0   No recall
1   Recalls odd incidents
2   Needs prompting
3   Memory intact

Social skills:
0   Disruptive
1   Offered nothing
2   Spoke only if asked
3   Responded only to staff
4   Responded to other members
5   Spontaneous

Participation:
0   No response
1   Unco-operative
2   Participated when asked
3   Actively participated

Pleasure:
0   No signs of pleasure
1   Occasionally showed pleasure
2   Enjoyed most of the session
3   Enjoyed all of the session
4   Gave pleasure to others

Concentration time:
0   Less than 5 minutes
1   5–10 minutes
2   10–20 minutes
3   Needed tuition
4   Mastered skill

Comments:

Fig. 12.12 Record of
activities.

> **RECORD OF ACTIVITY**
>
> Activity:
>
> Date: Time: Place:
>
> *Client's:*
>
> Eagerness to attend:
>
> Memory span:
>
> Social skills:
>
> Contribution:
>
> Pleasure:
>
> Equipment and materials used:
>
> Topics discussed:
>
> Themes and linked sessions:
>
> Liaison with other departments:
>
> Relatives involved:
>
> *Comments:*
>
> *Future events:*

Record writing

It is very important to record facts and to back these with examples from the event. Opinions are useful sometimes, but think about what you want to say, be sure you state it is an opinion and that it is backed with examples and facts. These opinions may be used as part of a decision about a person's ability to cope in various situations, or as part of a treatment package.

Do not be afraid of changing your opinion about a person. People change, especially clients meeting and functioning within a group. A person who appeared very confused and forgetful at first, may well progress surprisingly fast in the safe confines of a group. The regularity, same people and places helps the person to remember, the success of remembering gives confidence and improves ability in a variety of ways. This is not so for everybody, some clients find working with others confusing and do better in one to one situations. Whatever occurs, ensure that your records are accurate.

Summary

This chapter concentrates on clients as individuals and within a group, undertaking planned activities and events. Sessions are to help maintain both the mental and physical aspects of the client by encouraging memory and interaction and also improving manual dexterity and bodily strength.

There are many examples of activities that could be undertaken either in a client's home or within an activities unit under the supervision of a trained person. The careful 'matching' of a client with a specific activity is emphasized, along with individuality and choices made by the client, respecting their culture and dignity. Examples of charts are shown in order to keep accurate records for assessment and future planning.

This chapter considers and values the existing skills and the introduction of new interests and activities for the client, thereby enriching and adding purpose to their lives.

Further reading

Bettiss, C. (1993) Caution: music at work *Elderly Care*, July/August, **5**(1), 20.

Briscoe, T. (1991) Chapter 13, Activities, in Benson, S. & Carr, P. *Elderly Mentally Infirm People*. Care Concern Publication.

Bornat, J. (1994) *Reminiscence Reviewed*. Open University Press, Milton Keynes.

Clarke, A. & Hollands, J. (1996) *Leisure, Later Life and Homes*, Counsel & Care, London. Available from Counsel & Care, Twyman House, 16 Bonny Street, London NW1 9PG.

Coleman, P. (1986) *Ageing and Reminiscence Processes*. John Wiley, Chichesester.

Counsel and Care (1993) *Not Only Bingo*. Available from Counsel and Care. Twyman House, 16 Bonny Street, London NW1 9PG.

Ebersole, P. & Hess, P. (1993) *Towards Healthy Ageing*. C.V. Mosby, London.

Gibson, F. (1992) *The Reminiscence Handbook*. Age Exchange, The Reminiscence Centre, 11 Blackheath Village, London SE3 9LA.

Gibson, F. (1994) *Reminiscence and Recall: A Guide to Good Practice*. Available from Age Concern England, 1268 London Road, London SW16 4ER.

Gilley, J. & David, M. (1995) The living room. *Elderly Care*, May/June **7**(3), 9.

Holden, U. & Woods, R. (1982) *Reality Orientation*. Churchill Livingstone, London.

Hong, C. & Simmins, S. (1995) Linking past to present. *Elderly Care*, March/April, **7**(2), 9.

Marriott, V. & Timblick, T. (1988) *Loneliness: How to Overcome It*. Available from Age Concern, Astral House, 1268 London Road, London SW16 4ER.

Petre, T. (1996) Back into the swing of her social life. *Journal of Dementia Care*, January/February, **4**(1), 24.

Rigby, W. (1995) *Natural Therapies for Older People*. Hawker Publications, London.

Ruddlesden, M. (1995) *You Can Do It. Exercises for Older People*. Hawker Publications, London.

Walker, O. (1996) Music vibrates in the memory. *Journal of Dementia Care*, January/February **4**(1), 16.

Useful addresses

Recall tape slide series available from:
Help the Aged
St James's Walk,
London EC1R 0BE
Tel: 0171 253 0253

Bygone decades, nostalgia, memory
  jogger packs, available from:
Winslow Press
Telford Road
Bicester
Oxon OX6 0TS
Tel: 01869 244733

Making memories matter, books and
  packs from:
Age Exchange
The Reminiscence Centre
11 Blackheath Village
London SE3 9LA
Tel: 0181 318 9105

Section 5
Supporting Carers

Chapter 13
Caring for Carers
David Bell

Overview

This chapter focuses on the carers of older people. It discusses who they are; how to recognize their needs, how to involve them and support them. It looks at the feelings they may be experiencing and their relationships with the people they are caring for. The chapter also looks at how health care workers can increase their own satisfaction by helping carers to undertake clinical activities for the client and by enabling them to broaden their understanding of the client's needs and to support the client as changes are taking place.

Key words

Carers, partners, loss, bereavement, adjustment, coping with change, emotional support, practical support, information, partnership, interaction.

Definition of 'carer'

Carers are people who look after relatives or friends who, because of illness, disability or the effects of age, cannot manage at home without help. The life of a carer is restricted by the need to take responsibility for another person. The title *carer* can also be applied to friends or relatives who have in the past performed this role but are now visiting the person in a nursing or residential home. For the purposes of this chapter the term *care worker* will be used to describe professionals working with old people in the community, in hospitals or homes.

Do You Know?

There are probably 1.5 million people in Britain who are caring full-time for another person, and up to 7 million who care for over 20 hours a week (*The Observer* 1995). There are people of all ages and from every class and ethnic background acting as carers, and there is no typical person. However, 60 to 70% are women and their most likely age is between 48 and 64. Spouses, sons, daughters, grandchildren or neighbours can all take on the role. Services are becoming increasingly aware, for example, of young carers, many who still attend school, and the predicaments they face.

Carers are starting to be acknowledged by services. One estimate is that carers save up to £30 billion a year on health and social services expenditure by providing intensive social and nursing care to people who would otherwise have to be cared for in hospital or in residential or nursing homes. Social services now have to include an independent assessment of carers' needs when looking at clients' requirements (Levin and Moriarity, 1994).

The Carers (Recognition and Services) Act, 1995 and service planners have become increasingly sensitive to the feelings and needs of such a large number of people.

What happens to carers?

The carer may have been left in their role suddenly, following an accident or a 'traumatic' onset of illness.

Case study 1

Mrs Ryan suffered a disabling stroke at the age of 79. Her daughter, Anne, in her early 50s, was employed as a supervisor in a large department store. Anne and her husband lived very close to Mrs Ryan, but her sister and two brothers were all too distant to help very much. Anne's children had left home years before. At first Anne tried to carry on working, going to see her mother very early in the morning to get her up and give her breakfast, and going back as soon as she had finished work, but this was taking its toll on her, and her relationship with her husband was under stress. Her mother began having falls as she attempted to do things for herself unaided, and it was clear that she needed help throughout the day. Eventually Anne gave up her job, and would spend all day at her mother's home.

It was evident from this that her mother required considerable help. After Anne realized she was staying overnight in her mother's flat as well, sleeping on the sofa, she approached the local social services for her mother to be assessed.

The disability may have developed gradually, leaving the carer changing their role slowly over a period of time.

Case study 2

Mr Harris, since his retirement, had led an active life, walking the dog daily, spending time with his friends both in the pub and in the community centre. In the early years of his retirement his wife had accompanied him, but gradually seemed to become withdrawn and forgetful. She would be nervous in the company of people they had been close friends with and would not come out. As the years went by, the situation slowly deteriorated, with Mrs Harris saying uncharacteristic things, making accusations, and becoming depressed. Mr Harris' life became more and more centred around staying in with his wife, and when he did go out, he worried that she might leave the house and become lost or do something dangerous while he was away, such as turning on the gas and forgetting about it. Even at night Mrs Harris would awake and try to leave the house to 'go and find her mother'. Eventually the doctor enabled Mr and Mrs Harris to obtain a diagnosis of Alzheimer's Disease, and support was offered to them by the community psychiatric nurse and the local social services. By this time, though, Mr Harris had lost contact with many of his friends and had become tired and worried, a change in his own previous outlook on life.

Activity 13.1 ■■■■■■■■■■■■■■■■■■■■■■■■■■■■■

 Put yourself in the position of either of the carers in the examples given above. Make a list of the losses you would experience in the same situation.

■■■■■■■■■■■■■■■■■■■■■■■■■■■■■■■■■■

The following is by no means an exhaustive list, but some of the losses reported by carers include:

■ *Loss of income* perhaps having to claim benefits for the first time.
■ *Loss of employment* and of all that goes with a job: recognition, social contact, routine, self-esteem.
■ *Loss of independence* you may not be able to leave the person you care for, or at least have to think about them constantly while you are out.
■ *Loss of companionship* with the person you care for; you used to be very close, but they have changed, becoming depressed or angry and not good company anymore. You may no longer be able to discuss shared memories or plan a future, and sexual relationships may be very damaged.
■ *Loss of friends and family links* very often due to the difficulty of not knowing what to say or how to act with the disabled person, friends or other family members may stop visiting. This can lead to resentment from the carer, which can cloud the situation even further.
■ *Loss of sleep* sleep deprivation for the carers through disturbed nights on a regular basis can lead to increased stress in the short term and possible physical illness in the long term.

With all the above losses and with the other doubts and uncertainties that accompany the caring role – for example, embarrassment, feelings of guilt that you may be partly to blame for the illness or that you cannot do more for the person, lack of knowledge about the illness or of what to expect in the future – the experience of caring can be a very lonely one.

Loneliness can be a strong factor in developing depression. Carers not only have to give up their own life to care for another, but when it is no longer possible for the carer, for whatever reason, to continue and the dependant person is admitted to a nursing or residential home, the carer can be left with another level of loss – of their role as the most important person in the life of the dependant person. Also there is the loss of income that was related to that person, carers allowances or attendance allowance (refer to Chapter 7, Supported Living), and of the inter-dependence that may have developed over the years of committing themselves to one person. This needs to be acknowledged by staff working in hospitals or residential homes – for the benefit of the client, relative, or carer.

Activity 13.2 ■■■■■■■■■■■■■■■■■■■■■■■■■■■■■

 Think of a time when you have feelings similar to these. You may be a 'carer' yourself. Would you say you have ever 'cared for' someone, for example, a child, a parent or grandparent, or partner. Or you may have had to provide 'continuous care' for a client at work.

■■■■■■■■■■■■■■■■■■■■■■■■■■■■■■■■■■■■■

Types of support to offer carers or partners

It is clear that, with all the possible stresses and losses that carers experience, real support is sometimes needed from careworkers to help them to cope. The outcome of this support may help the client receive the highest quality care from both carers and care workers.

Carers normally report two main areas in which they need support. These areas can be categorized as:

■ *Emotional support* dealing with the feelings that come from their role as caring for a dependent person.
■ *Practical support* how to deal with the tasks they now have to perform for or with the person, and how to get access to information, both about the illness itself, and about the services or benefits to which they may be entitled. (Kubler-Ross, 1973)

Emotional support

Often the first area in which carers request help is the understanding by others of their own needs and situations.

For example, a daughter is talking to her mother, both are sitting in chairs in a corridor of the residential home. She asks her mother whether there is anything she needs from home. A voice comes from another room, 'She needs more cigarettes, and more knickers and a new pair of slippers – she wet the old ones!' It is the voice of a nurse who is making the bed inside the room.

Another example is a follows: a husband is sitting next to his wife in the early afternoon in the living room of the nursing home, his wife is dozing off and the husband, in his 80s, has nothing to do. Two nurses enter the room with a wheelchair and approach another resident – a frail lady of 84, who is also dozing. 'Come on Elsie, time to go to the toilet' they announce as they take one side each and virtually lift her into the wheelchair. The wheelchair has no footplates and is tipped backwards as the nurses leave the room. No acknowledgement is made of the other resident's husband, who has observed this with a look of anxiety on his face.

The above are examples of lack of support or understanding by the care worker of the carer's/relative's needs or worries, to say nothing of the attitude they reflect towards the client themselves. They are actually both reported incidents, and both incidents were raised as complaints with the managers of the homes. The feelings of clients who are living out their last years in an environment they have not chosen, and of family or friends who maintain contact with them require sensitivity on the part of the staff.

Helping the carer cope with loss

Thinking of the carer's experience as bereavement can be helpful in approaching the situation. There are generally accepted stages we all go through when we experience a bereavement. Different writers have described different stages in the process of coming to terms with death such as denial, anger, guilt, acceptance, though these stages do not necessarily happen in order and no two individuals are alike in the way that they cope with it (Rogers, 1951).

In practice, the most important thing for carers is that someone can acknowledge their bereavement. Providing a listening ear to their grief is a vital source of support. Carl Rogers described the quality most needed in this situation as 'empathy' – the ability to see the world as another person sees it. This is not the same as 'sympathy' which can be thought of as 'how I'd feel if the same thing happened to me'. Empathy involves taking a non-judgemental approach where the carer's feelings are acknowledged (refer to Chapter 2 Communications).

Activity 13.3 ■

 If you can, get together with two other colleagues. Try and give 20 minutes to carry out the following exercise. Spend three minutes talking to one of your colleagues about a particular topic for example, your last holiday. Get the third person to make notes on the listening skills that the listener used. Then change around and take it turns to play each of the parts, talker, listener, observer. This can be a very effective learning experience!

■ ■

Communication skills are more thoroughly outlined in Chapter 2 of this book, but to recap, here are a few of the listening skills you can use:

■ *Genuine, active listening* use clear and encouraging body language. For example, eye contact, but not staring, nodding, good use of 'personal space', relaxed but attentive pose.

■ *Open questions* questions that invite a fuller answer. For example 'How did it make you feel...?', 'What kind of things did you like to do...?' Be careful with questions, make sure you are confident enough to deal with the answers! Often we can release unexpected emotions by asking the simplest of questions!

■ *Use of silence* people do not stop thinking just because they have stopped talking. Give them time to finish before you fill the silence.

■ *Paraphrasing/reflecting* 'Let me see if I've understood this...' This has two benefits: first, you are letting the person know that you have been listening to what they have said, and second, you are checking that you have got it right.

■ *Stimulating the person to make suggestions* 'What would you have done if it had been you?' This helps them look at other ways of doing things.

These are just a few suggestions to help you hear what carers are saying, thus enabling them to realize that their feelings are valued.

Activity 13.4 ■

Ask a colleague to observe your next conversation with a client's relative. Ask them to discuss how you listened to the relative. Could you have been more encouraging, used body language to help the relative express themselves more clearly?

■ ■

Helping the carer deal with stress

There are anxieties that the carer may have lived with for years. In addition, increased worries raised by the need for the relative to go into hospital or residential or nursing home can leave them with a need for help in coping with the stress.

Activity 13.5 ■

Think back to the last time you faced a situation when you were in a strange place being observed and judged by others, for example your interview for your present job. Remember how it made you feel. Make a list of the signs that you noticed.

■ ■

Many people report a range of symptoms including tension, sweating, tightening of the stomach, shaking hands, a need to evacuate their bladder or bowel. All these are quite normal 'fight or flight' responses. They are part of animal behaviour to help us deal with what could be dangerous situations.

However, if these symptoms persist, they can become a problem. There has been much talk about the negative effects that long-term stress can have on your health. Sleep loss, migraines, increased sensitivity to infections, even ulcers are commonly reported. Everyone has their own way of coping with levels of stress: sport, exercise, listening to music, even cleaning the house! Others do not have very good strategies.

Three simple approaches, which can be easily suggested to carers who may not be coping very well with their own anxiety are described here.

(1) *Controlled breathing* concentrate on breathing slowly and count when stress symptoms are recognized.
(2) *Thought-switching* consciously replace maladaptive or negative self-talk, when we say to ourselves: 'I can't talk to that person – I'll find someone more friendly looking' with coping or positive statements: 'I can talk to them – they're only human!'
(3) *Relaxing the body* this needs to be done in a quiet environment where you feel private and safe. Many tapes are available now which give relaxation instructions, but an easy self-exercise is to carry out the following procedure:
   ■ Sit in a comfortable chair without arms, or lie on your back on the bed or on the carpet.
   ■ Start by closing your eyes and slowly – count to ten.
   ■ Tense all the muscles in your face, screwing your eyes up and clenching your jaw – count to ten.
   ■ Relax – count to ten.
   ■ Tense your neck and shoulders hunching them up to your ears – count to ten.
   ■ Relax – count to ten.
   ■ Hold out your arms with your fists clenched and tense them as hard as you are able – count to ten.
   ■ Relax – count to ten.

Repeat this procedure, remembering to count and relax, for all sets of muscles in your body. How do you feel at the end? This is a simple procedure which can be taught to carers to help them cope with immediate anxieties and stresses, enabling them to take a step back from the situation they are having difficulty with.

Activity 13.6 ■

Work with a colleague to practise basic relaxation techniques with you. Find a quiet room and a clear 15 minutes. Talk them through the relaxation exercise described above. Leave at least a few minutes at the end of the exercise for them to recover slowly. When you feel confident in the exercise, discuss with one of the carers/relatives you meet whether they may benefit from this.

■ ■

Acknowledging the carer's interpersonal needs

On admission to a residential or nursing home, the client can often experience a loss of independence, privacy and control over their own environment. They have to fit into a group living situation where they have not taken part in decisions made concerning how the home is organized. They have to follow the routines laid down for them by others: what time they eat, what time they go to bed; in some homes even visiting times are still limited.

This experience is very often the same for carers. At home they used to be the one who provided all the care, they decided with the dependent person what they would eat and when, if they needed to rest, what they could watch on television. They know their relative's likes and dislikes and why, they are able to be intimate with their relative or be angry, just as any normal human relationship. Once they become the visitor the situation has changed. They have to fit in with the routines of the home and very often see the home as belonging to the staff – as if it were someone else's territory. Intimacy and sexuality are areas of need which are rarely dealt with in residential settings. It is very difficult for staff to know how to approach them and for relatives to raise the subjects. Residential or nursing homes also need to incorporate an acknowledgement of the cultural and language needs of people from a variety of ethnic backgrounds.

One example of the 'alienation' of the carer is of the wife who is asked to wait in the day room while the care workers change her husband's wet clothes. The feelings she experiences might be of disempowerment, of guilt that she isn't able to help, of unspoken frustration that the staff treat her like this and of loss of self-esteem because she doesn't see a way of asking if she can help.

This is a difficult situation for care workers too. They feel that it is their job to carry out the tasks, they may feel under scrutiny and embarrassed if they performed the task in front of the relative, and they may feel that it is their territory. The situation can be improved by an open discussion with the relative.

Activity 13.7 ■

 Think of all the clients you work with. Are there any whose carers/relatives you feel confident in approaching to help in the tasks you carry out? Are they from a cultural or ethnic background different from the majority of the residents in the home? Is this addressed in their care plan?

■ ■

Carers need time to express how they are feeling about the admission of their relative to long-term care. For the majority, the decision to give up has been long and hard to make. They may have talked to other friends or family members about it, but unless they feel comfortable with the home and with the staff, they may continue feeling angry with themselves and ambivalent to the home. It is a sad fact that staff talk about difficult relatives. These tend to be people who ask about everything, are frequent visitors and show concern at every lost piece of clothing or change in their relative's condition. To improve the way carers feel about a home, we need to improve how we involve them from the beginning. On admission, they need to be consulted about everything to do with the client. This is becoming common practice in many homes, but there are many places where it is not. The more the staff know about the history, personality, likes and dislikes (not just of food but of clothing, activity, entertainment, etc.) and habits of the client, the easier the transition will be for the person concerned, for the staff and for the carer who has been involved with the whole admission process. The carer will have been shown by that process that they are valued by staff.

Finally, it is important to remember than not all relationships between people who have lived together for so many years are completely positive. Every home also has its fair share of relatives who never come and visit or clients who actively don't want particular people to come and visit them. Families are not all filled with caring relationships. There is a growing awareness in this society of the problems of elder abuse (refer to Chapter 6). There is also a possibility that the client may have treated the carer or relative badly in the past. This is information care workers may not be party to and it is advisable not to judge relatives who visit infrequently, or not at all, as uncaring.

Groups

Another very important way for carers to share their feelings about their own situation and about the home their relative is living in is by talking to other carers. This is also true for carers in the community as well. Many homes now have *relatives groups* which meet at varying frequencies. Groups provide an opportunity for carers to talk to others who have had similar if not the same experience as themselves. This chapter will not deal with the facilitating of groups such as this, but it must be emphasized that the sort of support that people in the same situation can offer each other is very often more meaningful and more lasting than anything that care staff, social workers, nurses or doctors can offer. This does not belittle what can be offered by professionals, but it has to be acknowledged that a shared situation, and a solution to a problem based on experience rather than what may be theory, can be more immediately helpful. Speakers can be invited to groups to discuss a large range of subjects which may support carers, services available, financial benefits and how to cope with particular problems.

Care workers can provide real support to individual carers by putting them in touch with support groups where they can share both problems and positive experiences. If there is not a group in the home that you work in, explore the possibility of setting up one with other staff, or research what groups may already be meeting in your area. Organizing and running groups is a skill that many care workers can and do develop.

Practical support

The second area reported by carers as a need for support is carrying out practical tasks for the dependent person. The carer may have looked after the relative on their own for a long time with little or no help. During this time, sometimes over many years, they have been used to carrying out varying degrees of nursing and social support. Often the last straw for the carer is the strain of the practical tasks involved in caring for someone with a high level of need. It is often at this point when the carer feels their relative should be in a nursing or residential home. Commonly reported 'last straws' include the increase of tasks for the carer in lifting, incontinence, eating difficulties, or specific confused behaviour such as wandering.

Either at home (in the community) or in a hospital ward, residential or nursing home, the benefits of staff carrying out practical or clinical tasks with carers and relatives are many.

Case study 3

Mr Briggs had worked as a doorman in a club after his retirement and was generally not back home until nearly midnight every night, after locking up. His wife developed a dementing illness fairly rapidly (becoming quite severe over three years). Her increasing disorientation, such as leaving the seventh floor flat at all hours because she had to 'go to school' or 'go home to her mother', left Mr Briggs with an impossible situation. Eventually, he had to give up his employment and subsequently became quite ill himself. The couple received input from a variety of sources, including relief carers and home helps. Much anxiety was raised when agency staff noticed that Mrs Briggs had bruising under her arms and on her knees. The worst was suspected, that Mr Briggs was maltreating his wife. However, Rose, one of the relief carers visiting the couple regularly, noticed that Mr Briggs would be the only one with his wife for the majority of the time and that he had to carry out tasks with her. These included encouraging Mrs Briggs in personal hygiene and helping her to stand to walk the short distance to the bedroom. Rose examined Mr Briggs' method of lifting his wife, which was far from safe for either of them, and reckoned that the bruising was probably a direct result of the husband's lack of training in this area. After talking to Mr Briggs about safe handling, Rose was able to demonstrate a method she had been taught of lifting and transferring a client. This proved easier for both husband and wife and no further bruising was reported.

Case study 4

Mr Davies, a retired docker, had suffered disability including a level of brain damage as a result of a road traffic accident at the age of 72. Mrs Davies, with the help of her family, had cared for him at home without a break for the last three years. He was admitted to a medical ward in a local hospital for investigations for incontinence. Staff found that he was very resistive when they were carrying out personal hygiene tasks with him and at meal times he would often lash out at the nurse who was trying to feed him. Consequently, his meals were rushed and he frequently went without adequate food. Mrs Davies had to fit into the visiting times and it wasn't until she approached several of the staff, and finally the ward manager, that she was invited to come in at meal times to help her husband eat and get washed and changed. This was of benefit to all parties, easing both Mr and Mrs Davies' anxieties.

Partnership

One of the practical areas that causes the greatest distress is that of incontinence. The highest level of distress is obviously for the clients themselves, but research into incontinence on wards or in nursing homes specifically, has identified the amount of staff time taken up by toileting – taking clients to the toilet every two or three hours and changing them between times when they are found to be wet (Norton & Fader, 1994). Refer to Chapter 9, Elimination.

More efficient interventions for incontinence are suggested but one such intervention can be to develop a *partnership* with the person who knows the client best: the carer or relative. Encouraged to participate in the planning of care for the client, they can be involved in visiting at particular times and they may recognize better than staff when the client needs to use the toilet. This may in the long run help maintain continence and reduce distress for both the carer and client. This is especially important if the stay in hospital is only temporary. Many carers complain that their relative had no problems prior to entering hospital, but was incontinent on discharge. A certain benefit of this approach is that it will help maintain the caring role and the sense of companionship.

The benefits of developing this partnership with carers are highlighted in case study 4. Lifting is a learned skill (refer to Chapter 11, Mobility), which needs to be approached very carefully. Carers often do know better than staff how to approach the client and how to get his or her co-operation to the full extent.

Eating difficulties

Another area of stress is in difficulties with *eating*. Staff often have difficulties in getting a client to eat, even after a full speech therapy assessment where there are no identifiable physical reasons for the problem. Clients may take a long time over a meal; some may refuse altogether. Many people with dementia, for example, have difficulty in recognizing objects placed in front of them or in initiating the activity of picking up a knife and fork to start the meal. Mutual understanding and co-operation between staff and carer can help the client. Staff can also help the carer understand some of the factors that lead to eating difficulties, perhaps perceptual or swallowing problems are involved (refer to Chapter, 8, Nutrition), carers can help by having more time when staff realistically are in the position that they need to give meals to a number of people in a short space of time. Carers usually know, more clearly, exactly what the client's likes and dislikes are. The experience in the second example above is very commonly reported.

Challenging behaviour

Dealing with *challenging behaviour* is another area where staff can improve the care for the client by sharing their experience with carers or relatives. Helping carers develop approaches to deal more calmly and patiently with confused or 'aggressive' behaviour can benefit all. Ward or nursing home staff can support carers in using the communication skills listed in Chapter 2 of this book. This may in itself alleviate much of the anxiety that precedes and stimulates challenging behaviour.

Carers or relatives often are prepared to be involved much more than they are allowed in the care of the client. Activities and outings are of vital importance in residential situations, and while there is a duty of care on the staff of the home, there is also a responsibility to provide a stimulating and satisfying life for the client (refer to Chapter 12, Leisure). Relatives who can be coached in lifting, use of mobility aids such as wheelchairs and improved methods of carrying out personal hygiene tasks with the client, are often the most supportive and satisfied (refer to Chapter 10, Hygiene, Comfort and Rest and Chapter 7, Supported Living).

Terminal illness

It is also vitally important to be aware of and sensitive to the needs and wishes of the carer during the terminal stages of illness. It is of paramount importance to decide with the carer or relative how much they wish to be involved in the palliative care of a dying patient. The religious and cultural customs and requirements of the client and carer must be respected. Care workers can make no assumptions, and every individual will deal with death in a different way. It is of vital importance for the client to be able to die in the company of those who care most for them with as much privacy as we can offer. If the *partnership of care* is not employed at this stage, there is a risk of increased stress and unresolved grief for the carer. Talk honestly to the carer about what is expected and allow them space to take as much part in the terminal care of a client as they wish.

It has to be remembered though, that there are times when carers, often due to lack of clear understanding or advice, have developed strategies for coping with practical difficulties in unorthodox ways. They may appear to be quite rough in the way they speak to a client or, as an example, in they way they physically handle their relative. Dealing with this requires sensitivity and understanding on the part of the staff and skill in approaching the issue honestly. If there is a doubt, care workers should discuss clearly with other staff the best way of approaching the situation. It can, however, be simply a matter of coaching (demonstrating to or working with) the carer to find an easier or more satisfactory method. Much of the time they will be happy to change their approach. It is often not until others tell us how we appear that we are able to perceive the results of our own behaviour (Fig. 13.1).

Overall, the client has to be the main benefactor of the partnership between carers and staff, but the general result of this approach is that frustrations and anxieties are reduced and everyone's life is made easier. All three parties must join forces to:

Fig. 13.1 Carer and care worker assisting client to stand.

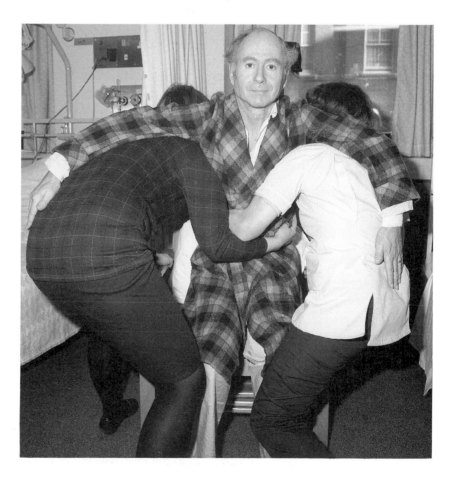

- Identify what difficulties are occurring
- Assess what the client's needs are
- Plan what interventions are to be made

to help clients achieve an improved quality of life (Figs 13.2 and 13.3)

Fig. 13.2 Carer and care worker identifying a care need.

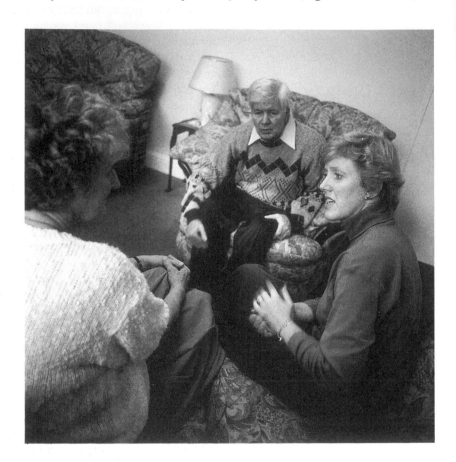

The need for information

Another very practical way in which carers want to be supported by staff is in gaining access to information. This is an area where clearly the balance of power in the care worker/carer relationship is weighted against the carer. All reports of carer's needs state that they would like clearer information in a range of areas:

- The illness/disability itself – what caused it, what to expect in the future.
- What the treatments are doing for the person – how medications work, what side-effects there are.

■ How to deal with particular difficulties related to the specific disability – e.g. speech and language difficulties in stroke, *tardive dyskinesia* in Parkinson's Disease, the failure of face recognition in Alzheimer's Disease.

■ What services are available to support carers from all sources – such as home support from social services, respite care from Cross-roads, visits from district nurses. Carers are very often unclear about (sometimes completely baffled by) what help they are entitled to, who provides it and how to get access to it (refer to Chapter 7, Supported Living).

■ What financial benefits they may be entitled to as a carer, or what the client may be able to claim such as council tax relief, invalid care allowance, attendance allowance, taxi cards, etc.

This can be a very difficult area to deal with. Information can be offered in many different ways but careful work with clients can identify what they need. Carers want information, but how do staff know exactly what information the carers need, and how simple or in-depth should the information be? How many times has a specialist like a car mechanic or a plumber explained what they have done without checking that you have grasped what they are describing?

The care worker needs to be able to use their listening skills to be able to hear clearly what difficulties the carer is experiencing and put across useful information in a way that is accessible, friendly and not patronizing. They need to use language that is geared towards the individual carer's situation.

Fig. 13.3 Giving instructions as to how to carry out care.

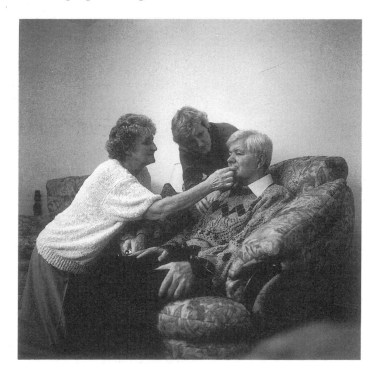

Activity 13.8 ■■■■■■■■■■■■■■■■■■■■■■■■■■■■■■■

Think about the clients in your care. Make a list of their illnesses/disabilities. Spend time with a colleague explaining the main features of the diagnosis. Has your colleague understood. Make a point of filling in the gaps.

■■■■■■■■■■■■■■■■■■■■■■■■■■■■■■■■■■■■

Activity 13.9 ■■■■■■■■■■■■■■■■■■■■■■■■■■■■■■■

List your interactions with carers or relatives over the last two weeks. Can you think of any area where practical or emotional support offered to the carers or relatives may have improved their understanding of a situation or enabled the client to receive better quality care?

■■■■■■■■■■■■■■■■■■■■■■■■■■■■■■■■■■■■

Activity 13.10 ■■■■■■■■■■■■■■■■■■■■■■■■■■■■■■

Get together with a colleague at your place of work. Make a list of any ways in which carers/relatives could be made to feel more involved in the care of the client in your place of work.

■■■■■■■■■■■■■■■■■■■■■■■■■■■■■■■■■■■■

You could mention:

- Making carers feel welcome and involved during the admission procedure
- Gathering information from them
- Specifically spending a little time with them each day to talk about themselves and how things have been with the client
- Putting carers in touch with a group or getting them to help in particular practical tasks or clinical procedures with the client.

Summary

Traditionally the *caring relationship* has existed either between the carer and client at home, or between the care worker and client, nurse/patient in the hospital or nursing home. The growth in understanding of the carer's situation and the real benefits that good communication with the carer and quality support that the carer can offer to the client have changed that.

Our emphasis now has to be on *partnership* and *interaction*. There is now a clearer understanding that if older clients, carers and care workers communicate well and work together, the experience of illness or disability, whether in the hospital, nursing home or in the community, can be improved for all.

References

Norton & Fader (1994) Incontinence. *Elderly Care*, November/December **6** (6) 23.

Kubler-Rose, E. (1973) *On Death and Dying*. Tavistock Publications, London.

Levin & Moriarty (1994) *Better For The Break*. National Institute of Social Work Research Unit. HMSO, London.

Rogers, C. (1951) *Client-Centred Therapy*. Constable, London.

The Observer (1995) One in nine. *The Observer*, 7 May.

Further reading

Age Concern (1995) *Your Rights – A Guide to Benefits for Retired People*. Age Concern, London.

Bowlby, J. (1980) *Loss*. Penguin, London.

Carers Association (1994) *Carers Code: Eight Key Principles for Health and Social Care Providers*. Available from, Carers National Association, 20–25 Glasshouse Yard, London EC1A 4JS.

Corti, L. *et al.* (1995) Informal carers and employment. *Employers Gazette*, March, available from Scottish Council for Voluntary Organisations, 18–19 Claremont Crescent, Edinburgh EH7 5QD.

Crompton, S. (1995) *The Carers Guide to Essential Information for People Looking After Others*, 2nd edn. Macmillan, London.

Forster, M. (1989) *Have the Men Had Enough?* Penguin, London.

Gilleard, C.J. (1984) *Living with Dementia*. Croomhelm Ltd, Beckenham.

Gilleard, C.J. & Watt, G. (1983) *Coping with Ageing Parents*. MacDonald Ltd, Loanhead, Midlothian.

Holden, U. *et al.* (1980) *24 Hour Approach to the Problem of Confusion in Elderly People*. Winslow Press, Bicester.

Kingston, P. & Penhale, B. (1995) (eds) *Family Violence and Caring Professions*. Macmillan, London.

Lodge, B. (1981) *Coping with Caring – a Guide to Identifying and Supporting an Elderly Person with Dementia*. Mind, London.

Mace, N.L. & Rabins, P.V. (1985) *The 36 Hour Day*. Hodder & Stoughton, London.

Mawby, D. (1993) Support for the carers. *Nursing Times*, 9 June **89** (23), 67.

Murphy, P. & Kupscik, G.A. (1992) *Loneliness and Stress and Well-being*. Routledge, London.

Orton, C. (1989) *Care for the Carer*, Thorsons, an Imprint of Harper Collins Publishers, London.

Scottish Health Board (1995) *Keeping Safe a Guide to Safety When Someone Lives Alone*. Available from Scottish Health Board, Woodburn House, Canon Lane End, Edinburgh EH10 4SG, Scotland.

Thomas, S. (1993) Lessons to be learnt, *Nursing Times*, 30 June **89** (26), 38.

Useful addresses

Alzheimer's Disease Society
2nd floor, Gordon House
Greencoat Place
London SW1 1PH

Boots Carers
PO Box 94
Nottingham NG2 3AA
or
Boots Carers Hotline
Tel: 0602 592 282
For free copy of *Fair Deal for Carers – A Carer's Guide to Getting Services*

Carers' National Association
Ruth Pitter House
20/25 Glasshouse Yard
London EC1A 4JS

Cross-roads
Information and details:
Yvonne McCann
Tel: 01788 573 653

National Association of Adult Placement Services (NAAPS)
51a Rodney Street
Liverpool L1 9ER
Tel: 0151 709 1200
For information concerning a specialist scheme for public liability insurance cover

NAAPS, TaxAid
Tel: 0151 624 3768
For TaxAid booklet, information also available from any Inland Revenue inquiry
offices concerning income tax allowances for professional carers

The National Carers Association (England)
29 Chilworth Mews
London W2 3RG

The National Carers Association (Scotland)
11 Queen's Cresent
Glasgow G4 9AS

The Princess Royal Trust for Carers
Tel: 0171 480 7788 for your nearest Carers Centre

Accreditation of Prior Learning

Kate Arter

Introduction

It is likely that many health care workers reading this book have been involved in caring for older people for some time – some perhaps for many years. They may have gained a great deal of job satisfaction, but will probably have received no formal recognition for the skills and knowledge they have acquired. Accreditation of Prior Learning, or APL, as it is known, is a process whereby an individual can present evidence of past experience to demonstrate that they meet the standard defined in National Vocational Qualifications (NVQs) or Scottish Vocational Qualifications (SVQs). Many approved assessment centres offer APL support to S/NVQ candidates. This appendix introduces the APL route to gaining a qualification.

It will guide health care workers as follows:

■   Suitability
■   Outline the process
■   Suggest the forms that evidence can take
■   Advise on how to obtain support if they wish to proceed

The APL route

APL recognizes that people learn from their experience, and that skills and knowledge gained in this way are of equal value to those gained in a formal educational setting. Evidence to prove their achievements can therefore be assessed independently of any traditional learning programme.

There are broadly five distinct stages to the APL process:

(1)   Identifying and reviewing the skills and knowledge achieved
(2)   Matching these to S/NVQ units of competence
(3)   Gathering evidence into a portfolio to prove competence
(4)   Assessment of the evidence
(5)   Being certificated with the S/NVQ, or credit towards one, together with receiving guidance and feedback

It is most important to remember that even though evidence from the past may be included in the portfolio, this must demonstrate that a carer is *currently* competent. Any skill acquired demands continued practice to maintain it, whether it be 70 words-per-minute touch typing, wind surfing or giving skilled care to clients! The process is illustrated diagrammatically in Fig. App1.1

Fig. App1.1 The APL process.

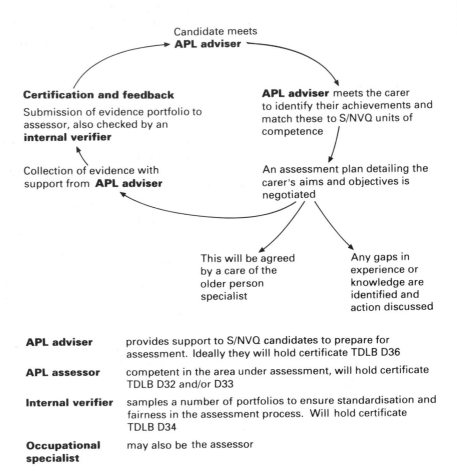

APL adviser	provides support to S/NVQ candidates to prepare for assessment. Ideally they will hold certificate TDLB D36
APL assessor	competent in the area under assessment, will hold certificate TDLB D32 and/or D33
Internal verifier	samples a number of portfolios to ensure standardisation and fairness in the assessment process. Will hold certificate TDLB D34
Occupational specialist	may also be the assessor

Advantages of APL

The first stage of APL, identifying and reviewing existing skills and knowledge, can be enormously morale-boosting, particularly for those with little formal educational background. In this alternative route to qualifications, carers can work at their own pace with no requirement to attend a formal college course. It encourages carers to take responsibility for their own development while enhancing self-esteem and career prospects. The portfolio of evidence developed is a most useful aspect which can be discussed at job interviews, or when seeking admission to higher education. Areas where an individual is weak can be identified and the national S/NVQ standards will help a carer to ascertain any training and development needs and plan how these can be met. Often these are small gaps in knowledge which can be addressed by a visit to a library or indeed by this book!

S/NVQs recognize competence in the workplace and APL is a cost-effective way to achieve this recognition. Employers will be pleased. S/NVQs enable organizations and clients to be confident in the skills of staff and are, in themselves, highly motivating.

For whom is APL suitable?

There are a variety of routes to gain an S/NVQ, and APL is a particularly suitable one for people who are *motivated* to achieve recognition for their skills. They need to have *practised recently* and must have a *range of experience* in order to meet the full requirements of one of the qualifications aimed at those who care for older people. It is suitable for those who have qualifications gained overseas and which are not recognized in the UK, or for those who have gained a qualification such as a BTEC First in Caring which has given them a good grounding, but does not prove their competence in the way an S/NVQ does.

Prospective APL candidates need to have good organizational skills, a realistic self-image and feel comfortable with writing. It is helpful if they have access to support from their colleagues, employer, family or fellow APL candidates.

Candidates can use APL to gain one or more units of competence, but if they wish to achieve the entire qualification it is ideal if they already have the bulk of their evidence to build into a portfolio.

APL is more difficult for . . .

The self-employed, those lacking in confidence and carers needing a lot of top-up training.

APL is not suitable for . . .

Those with little or narrow work experience, those with no spare time and those who need constant external motivation.

An APL advisor will offer the support needed to decide!

The APL process

Identify and review achievements

There are currently 20 S/NVQs in care and a number of endorsements suitable for those who care for older people. Taking a care worker's role as a starting point helps to clarify their responsibilities, the skills and knowledge required to meet them and identify the most suitable qualification to aim for. 'Mind mapping' is a useful technique to use. A large piece of paper is required! The simplified map of one care worker's role is shown in Fig. App1.2.

Fig. App1.2 A simplified 'mind map' of a care assistant's role.

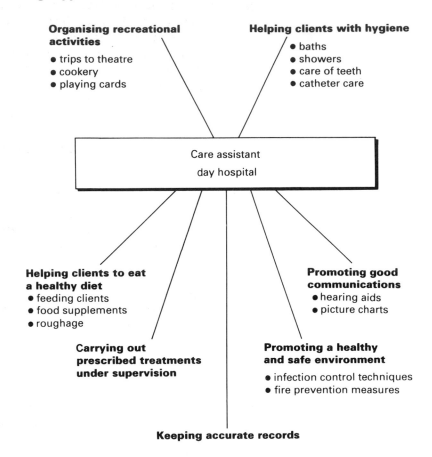

Organising recreational activities
- trips to theatre
- cookery
- playing cards

Helping clients with hygiene
- baths
- showers
- care of teeth
- catheter care

Care assistant
day hospital

Helping clients to eat a healthy diet
- feeding clients
- food supplements
- roughage

Carrying out prescribed treatments under supervision

Promoting good communications
- hearing aids
- picture charts

Promoting a healthy and safe environment
- infection control techniques
- fire prevention measures

Keeping accurate records

Activity App1.1 ■

 Start to map your responsibilities in the same way. You will be able to think of many more than those illustrated in Fig. App1.2. This will be very useful and will save time when you meet your APL advisor.

■ ■

It may help to discuss this with a manager or a colleague, who may suggest additional responsibilities.

Matching achievements to NVQ units of competence

The APL advisor will help the carer to identify the units in which they are already competent. The advisor may do this through discussion, using a skill scan or check-list, checking out the breadth of experience the carer has in the areas of responsibility they identified as in Activity App1.1 above.

Having identified the units of competence in which the carer is already competent, the advisor and care worker will negotiate an assessment plan and consider the ways in which the carer can prove their competence. At the start of the process it is advisable to focus on one unit, and analyse experience in detail. The S/NVQ standards should be referred to. They describe the range of situations in which competencies must be demonstrated and the *performance criteria* specify the standard to be achieved. The S/NVQ standards also give guidance on the evidence required and detail the knowledge needed to underpin performance.

Sometimes it works best to approach this on a unit basis, however when a unit is very diverse it is advisable to take each element separately.

Building an evidence portfolio

The term 'evidence' has been used frequently in this chapter so far, but what forms can this evidence of competence take? The key here is to be imaginative and think laterally. The evidence may be described as direct or indirect.

Direct evidence

This is generated by the care worker – something they have done, made or undertaken during their normal job role. Here are some examples of direct evidence

- Letters
- Memos
- Kardex
- Diary entries
- Requisitions
- Records

- Photographs
- Video recordings
- Tape recordings
- Any other work products, such as a communication aid made by the carer

Another important point: remember to ensure that confidentiality of clients is maintained. The rule is that no-one should be able to recognize a client from reading a portfolio of evidence. This can be achieved by the use of either pseudonyms or white correction fluid! When this is not necessarily approp.iate or possible, for example when using photographs as evidence, then the client's permission should be sought beforehand.

Indirect evidence

This is used to describe your achievements, for example:

- Testimonies by clients, managers, colleagues, etc. confirming your claim for competence and authenticating evidence
- Certificates awarded as a result of tests or examinations

- Case studies
- Storyboards or accounts of how procedures or situations are approached, or, describing how the demands of the value base unit are met
- Details of training courses you have attended

Evidence can also be generated by demonstrating competence to, or answering questions posed by, an assessor in the care worker's workplace. This will need to be described by the assessor in writing for inclusion in the portfolio. The same evidence can be used in a number of different ways to demonstrate competence in several units and elements. The approved assessment centre will guide the carer as to how best to cross-reference evidence.

The assessment of the portfolio of evidence by an APL assessor is likely to include an interview during which the carer will be asked questions. Anything that has not been made sufficiently clear can be clarified at this time.

Activity App 1.2 ■

Figure App 1.3 below is a 'mind map' detailing the range to be addressed in one unit of competence: unit Z13 – Enable clients to participate in recreation and leisure activities. Underneath each range statement suggest evidence that you have generated, or could generate, which would prove you meet the standards outlined in the performance criteria and that you have the knowledge required to underpin your performance. You will need to demonstrate that you collected the evidence while working with three different clients.

■ ■

Note how the two elements in the unit have been combined so that you can link together evidence about the *planning* of the activity with evidence about how you provided *support* to the clients while they undertook the activity.

Here are some suggestions:

- Photographs or a video recording taken during a visit to the coast organized by the care worker (non-sedentary, group activity, outside the care setting) combined with a report on how the care worker approached this and the differing factors to be taken into account before such a trip could be undertaken (knowledge and supporting evidence).
- A number of small case studies detailing how the care worker helped clients to enjoy pastimes of their choice, within the care setting (sedentary, individual activity, within care setting). An explanation of how the care worker accommodated their likes and dislikes and helped to overcome any disability should be included (knowledge and

supporting evidence). A testimony from the manager, authenticating the care worker's role in these case studies, would be important indirect evidence.

Fig. App1.3 Action plan for Unit Z13, detailing range to be assessed.

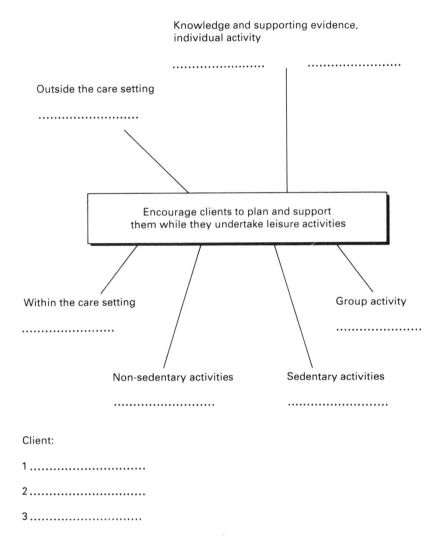

Z13 Enable clients to participate in recreational and leisure activities

Knowledge and supporting evidence, individual activity

....

Outside the care setting

....

Encourage clients to plan and support them while they undertake leisure activities

Within the care setting

....

Group activity

....

Non-sedentary activities

....

Sedentary activities

....

Client:

1 ....

2 ....

3 ....

As the evidence is gathered together into a portfolio, it is important to reflect on its content. Asking the following questions will help to ensure a successful outcome.

■ Is the evidence *valid*? Does it relate closely to the unit of competence? Does it cover all the performance criteria and the range?
■ Is it *authentic*? Does it prove *current* competence? Could the care worker undertake the work to the required standard *today*?

■ Is there sufficient evidence? Does it cover the required number of clients, situations, etc. as demanded by the standards?
■ Is there any additional evidence which could be generated?

Assessment of the evidence

The portfolio of evidence will be assessed by an assessor who is competent in the caring of older people. The assessor will read the portfolio to ensure that every unit, element, performance criteria and range statement is addressed and that the evidence demonstrates that the required standards have been met. They may wish to interview the care worker and a tape of this interview would provide additional evidence. Parts of the portfolio will also be checked by an internal verifier and may even be seen by an external verifier appointed by the awarding body (City and Guilds of London Institute, Business and Technology Education Council or the Central Council for Education and Training in Social Work). Assessing the portfolio is a very rigorous business!

Certification guidance and feedback

The assessor will inform the care worker in which units they have achieved the competence standards and, for these, certificates of unit credit will be given. If and when all the units are achieved, then the S/NVQ certificate will be awarded.

For any units where the standards have not been met, guidance will be given as to any further evidence, learning or experience needed.

Further information

For details of approved assessment centres, the three awarding bodies who offer S/NVQs in Care will be able to help. These are:

City and Guilds of London Institute
1 Giltspur Street
London EC1A 9DD
Tel: 0171 294 2468

Business and Technology Education Council
Central House
Upper Woburn Place
London WC1H 0HH
Tel 0171 413 8400

Central Council for Education and Training in Social Work
Derbyshire House
St Chad's Street
London WC1H 8AD
Tel: 0171 278 2455

The local Training and Enterprise Council will know of centres that offer APL. It may also offer financial support as a contribution to the cost.

The Inland Revenue Vocational Tax Relief scheme enables care workers to receive a 25% discount on registration and recording fees of an S/NVQ. It is worth enquiring about this from the approved assessment centre.

Summary

It is hoped that this introduction to APL has enabled some readers to recognize the value of the skills and knowledge they already have and how evidence of their competence can be certificated without the need to attend course or study days, unless these have been identified as a real need. The increased confidence and sense of achievement that results from gaining an S/NVQ, especially through the APL route, will be ample reward for the time and effort needed to build the evidence portfolio. Good luck!

Further reading

Whitear, G. (1995) *The NVQ and GNVQ Handbook and Guide to Career Success*. Pitman Publishing, London.

Cross-reference with NVQ/SVQ units of competence for the Care awards
Christine McMahon

The contents of this book are cross-referenced with specific units of competence that primarily reflect the care of the older person. Units will be found for both level 2 and 3 Care awards and include some of the core units.

The underpinning knowledge for the units is covered, but as each chapter is not a definitive work, a list of suggested further reading will be found at the end of each of these. It should be possible to find this information in your local library or within the library of a Further or Higher College of Education or a College of Nursing.

Addresses are also included of many groups who circulate relevant information on the care of the older person.

Unit of competence/element Core at levels 2 and 3	Chapter
O unit Promote equality for all individuals	
This is reflected on all chapters, and primarily in the following:	
(a) Promote anti-discriminatory practice	3, 4, 5, 6, 7, 8, 9, 10
(b) Maintain confidentiality of information	2, 3, 4
(c) Promote and support individuals' rights and choices within a service delivery	4, 5, 6, 7, 8, 9, 10, 11, 12, 13
(d) Acknowledge individuals' personal beliefs and identity	2, 3, 4, 5, 6, 7, 8, 9, 10, 12, 13
(e) Support individuals through effective communication	2, 3, 5, 6, 7, 8, 9, 10, 12, 13
Z1 *Contribute to the protection of individuals from abuse*	6, 13
Z3 *Contribute to the management of aggressive and abusive behaviour*	2, 13

Unit of competence/element Core at levels 2 and 3	Chapter
Z4 *Promote communication with clients where there are communication difficulties*	2, 3
Z8 *Support clients when they are distressed*	2, 3
Y2 *Enable clients to make use of available services and information*	7, 13
W2 *Contribute to the ongoing support of clients and others significant to them*	2, 3, 13
W3 *Support clients in transition due to their care requirements*	13
U4 *Contribute to the health safety and security of individuals of individuals and their environment*	9, 10, 11

Unit of competence/element Endorsement units at levels 2 and 3	Chapter
Z2 *Contribute to the provision of advocacy for clients*	5
Z5 *Enable clients to move within their environment*	7, 11
Z6 *Enable clients to maintain and improve their mobility*	11
Z7 *Contribute to the movement and treatment of clients to maximize their physical comfort*	10, 11
(a) Prepare the client and environment for moving and lifting	11
(b) Assist the client to move from one position to another	11
(c) Assist the client to prevent and minimize adverse effects of pressure	10, 11
Z9 *Enable clients to maintain their personal hygiene and appearance*	7, 10
Z10 *Enable clients to eat and drink*	8
Z11 *Enable clients to access and use toilet facilities*	7, 9
Z12 *Contribute to the management of client continence*	9
Z13 *Enable clients to participate in recreation and leisure activities*	12, 13

Unit of competence/element Endorsement units at levels 2 and 3	Chapter
Z14 *Support clients and others at times of loss*	1, 13
Z18 *Support clients where abuse has been disclosed*	6
Z19 *Enable clients to achieve physical comfort*	10
Y1 *Enable clients to manage their domestic and personal resources*	7, 13
Y2 *Enable clients to make use of available services and information*	7, 13
Y3 *Enable clients to administer their financial affairs*	7, 13
Y4 *Support clients and carers in undertaking health care for the client*	13
Y5 *Assist clients to move from a supportive to an independent living environment*	7, 13
X1 *Contribute to the support of clients during developmental programmes and activities*	12, 13
X2 *Prepare and provide agreed individual development activities for clients*	12
W1 *Support clients in developing their identity and personal relationships*	3, 5
W4 *Assist occupational therapists in the provision of support and equipment to clients and carers in the community*	7
W5 *Support clients with difficult or potentially difficult relationships*	3, 5
W8 *Enable clients to maintain contacts in potentially isolating situations*	7
V1 *Contribute to the planning and monitoring of a service delivery*	2, 4
V2 *Determine ways in which the service can support clients*	4, 13
U1 *Contribute to the maintenance and management of domestic and personal resources*	7, 8, 10, 13
(a) Maintain a supply of personal clothes and linen	7, 10
(e) Prepare food and drink for clients	8

Index